Neurophysiology

Picture to yourself a scheme of lines and nodal points gathered together at one end into a great raveled knot, the brain, and at the other tailing off to a sort of stalk, the spinal cord. Imagine activity in this shown by little points of light. Of these some stationary points flash rhythmically, faster or slower. Others are traveling points streaming in serial lines at various speeds. The rhythmic stationary lights lie at the nodes. The nodes are both goals whither converge, and junctions whence diverge, the lines of traveling lights. Suppose we choose the hour of deep sleep. Then only in some sparse and out-of-the-way places are nodes flashing and trains of light points running. The great knotted head-piece lies for the most part quite dark. Occasionally at places in it lighted points flash or move but soon subside.

Should we continue to watch the scheme, we should observe after a time an impressive change which suddenly accrues. In the great head end, which had been mostly darkness, spring up myriads of lights, as though activity from one of these local places spread far and wide. The great top-most sheet of the mass, where hardly a light had twinkled or moved, becomes now a sparkling field of flashing points with trains of traveling sparks hurrying hither and thither. It is as if the Milky Way entered upon some cosmic dance. Swiftly the head mass becomes an enchanted loom where millions of flashing shuttles weave a dissolving pattern, always a meaningful pattern though never an abiding one. The brain is waking and with it the mind is returning.

Sir Charles Sherrington

This version of a passage by Sherrington, reprinted with permission, is quoted from Wilder Penfield in his chapter, "The Physiological Basis of Mind," in *Control of the Mind,* a symposium edited by S. M. Farber and R. H. L. Wilson (San Francisco, 1961, McGraw-Hill [pp. 4–5]). A slightly different version of the passage is provided by J. C. Eccles and W. C. Gibson in *Sherrington: His Life and Thought* (Berlin, 1979, Springer International [p. 122]), as a quoted excerpt from Sherrington's seventh lecture in the Gifford Lecture series at Edinburgh University in 1937. Sherrington uses an elaborated version of the passage in his book, *Man on his Nature,* published in New York by the Macmillan Company in 1941 (pp. 223-225).

Neurophysiology

James E. Blankenship, PhD
Ashbel Smith Professor
Marine Biomedical Institute and Departments of Anatomy and
    Neurosciences and Physiology and Biophysics
University of Texas Medical Branch
Galveston, Texas

 Mosby

An Affiliate of Elsevier Science
St. Louis   London   Philadelphia   Sydney   Toronto

Mosby

An Affiliate of Elsevier Science

The Curtis Center
Independence Square West
Philadelphia, Pennsylvania 19106

NOTICE

Medicine is an ever-changing field. Standard safety precautions must be followed, but as new research
and clinical experience broaden our knowledge, changes in treatment and drug therapy may become
necessary or appropriate. Readers are advised to check the most current product information provided by the manufacturer of each drug to be administered to verify the recommended dose, the
method and duration of administration, and contraindications. It is the responsibility of the licensed
prescriber, relying on experience and knowledge of the patient, to determine dosages and the best
treatment for each individual patient. Neither the publisher nor the editor assumes any liability for any
injury and/or damage to persons or property arising from this publication.

International Standard Book Code 0-323-01899-8

Acquisitions Editor: Jason Malley
Developmental Editor: Kevin Kochanski
Publication Services Manager: Patricia Tannian
Senior Project Manager: Anne Salmo
Senior Book Design Manager: Gail Morey Hudson
Cover Design: Rokusek Design

RT/QWF

Printed in the United States of America

Last digit is the print number: 9 8 7 6 5 4 3 2 1

Preface

This book is written to help the beginning student gain an understanding of the basic principles and processes that underlie the electrophysiological properties of nerve cells—how neurons produce the electrical potentials that are a hallmark of neural activity. The material is presented in a format that has proven helpful to many medical and graduate students whom I have taught over the years. The book is not meant to be comprehensive or exhaustive in its treatment of the topics covered but rather to be thorough and clear in its explanations and descriptions. It has been my experience that many students come to the subject of "electrical properties of nerve cells" with some trepidation and wariness: they are afraid the material is going to be too complicated or difficult. It does not have to be that way, and I hope you will agree after using this book.

It is assumed that the reader has had some basic chemistry, physics, and possibly cell biology, but you do not need to be an electrical engineer or math whiz to get the fundamental concepts. I have pushed the mathematical equations, electrical circuitry, and physical chemistry only so far. More advanced texts deal with the details and subtleties.

The first chapter provides a broad overview of the material. Subsequent chapters cover the properties, origins, and functions of resting potentials, action potentials, electrotonic behavior of membranes, and synaptic connections. Chapters 2 to 7 include questions that are inserted in the text and at the end of each chapter. You are encouraged to answer these questions as they appear. The questions are designed to help you understand and review the material and to reinforce assimilation of the information. If you find the questions distracting or interruptive, skip them. But answering the questions as you go will help you grasp and retain the basic ideas better. Getting a firm grip on this material does take some effort, so work your way through deliberately and thoroughly. You will soon discover that the information is not scary or incomprehensible—it is fascinating! Nerve cells really are remarkable; ensembles of nerve cells are astonishing; nervous systems are miracles.

The framework and approach used for this material owes much to David Potter, Edwin Furshpan, John Nicholls, and their colleagues who created the curriculum for a new Neurobiology Department at Harvard many years ago. I am grateful for the care and insight they provided in developing a coherent, organized, and inspiring pedagogy that made neurobiology both understandable and appealing. I remember being part of standing ovations by medical and graduate students at Yale for John Nicholls' lectures on these topics. Many of my own notes from that era formed the core on which I have developed some of these chapters. In more recent years I have learned from another gifted teacher and friend, Bill Willis, who as a superb scholar and able department chair has supported and encouraged excellent teaching.

v

My secretary, Ms. Lonnell Simmons, has provided an invaluable service in helping prepare this book, and I am most grateful. The best help and advice I have received, however, have come from students. Their feedback and constructive criticism honed the treatment significantly. It is their encouragement that lets me hope that this book may help other students beginning the fascinating journey into neurobiology.

James E. Blankenship

To
Patrick, Jack, Siera, Mollie, and **Ellie,**
who have had their own ways of teaching me

Contents

Contents

Neurophysiology

CHAPTER 1

Introduction and Overview

■ NERVE CELLS USE ELECTRICAL POTENTIALS AND THEIR EXTRAORDINARY SHAPES TO CREATE A COMMUNICATIONS SYSTEM

Neurophysiology is the study of how nerve cells (neurons) function, and the main function of neurons is to produce meaningful electrical signals. Several types of electrical "signals" are introduced here and elaborated on in successive chapters. This book will help you understand where these electrical signals come from and how they work. The way in which neurons create and utilize electrical signals is a unique property of these cells, although other cells such as skeletal, cardiac and smooth muscle fibers, and supportive cells of the brain (glial cells) have some, comparatively limited electrical signaling capabilities. Neurons also have another unique property—their extraordinary and complex morphology (Figure 1-1). The physical shape of a neuron, the geometric dimensions of its processes, and the contacts it makes with other neurons profoundly influence how that neuron functions and are as important to the integrity of the nervous system as the biochemical and electrical properties of neurons. Neurons work by being part of a "system," whether that system is the human brain with perhaps 100 billion individual nerve cells or a simple invertebrate neural ganglion with a few thousand neurons. Neurons work as individual members of groups of cells that signal one another to process sensory information or carry out motor and behavioral acts— to underlie virtually everything we do. Thus nerve cells are distinguished from other cell types for three important reasons: (1) they generate a variety of electrical signals, (2) they have specialized shapes and processes, cytoplasmic extensions from the cell body, more elaborate and complex than any other cell type, and (3) they make functional connections (synapses) among themselves and with target cells such as glands and muscles. The extensive network of processes and synaptic interactions are two aspects of the same basic feature: *connectivity*. Thus bioelectricity and functional connectivity (where and how neural processes interact) are the hallmark characteristics of neurons.

This insight was not casually derived. At the turn of the century the prevailing thought was that nervous tissue was a kind of syncytium. Nerve cells were believed to be in cytoplasmic continuity with one another, and the brain was seen as an interconnected mass of nuclei and

1

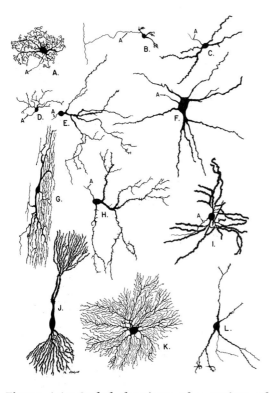

Figure 1-1 ■ Scaled drawings of a variety of representative neurons from different parts of the central nervous system of the monkey. Note the elaborate dendritic trees and the single axon *(A)* emanating from the soma. (From Carpenter MB, Sutin J: *Human neuroanatomy*, ed 8, Baltimore, 1983, Williams & Wilkins, p. 94.)

cytoplasmic extensions influencing one another through protoplasmic bridges. The remarkable work of the Spanish neuroanatomist, Ramón y Cajal, revolutionized our view of brain tissue. His systematic, precise, and prodigious work of interpreting stained nervous tissue clearly demonstrated that nerve cells, regardless of their complex and delicate shapes, are structurally individual entities. They make contiguous connections with one another (it took the electron microscope to see how really close the membranes of nerve cells come to one another), but they are not

in protoplasmic continuity. Thus the nervous system is composed of individual nerve cells; this is the *neuron doctrine*. This doctrine may seem obvious in hindsight, but it was once a raging controversy and symbolized more than a simple anatomical observation. It meant that we could move from a mystical view of brain as a paste-like mass of jelly with almost ethereal, meta-physical attributes to a brain of well-defined subunits, with order and biological properties amenable to systematic analysis.

The integration of information and execution of complex functions by neural circuits require myriad interconnections among nerve cells, and to accommodate this it was advantageous for neurons to elaborate their shape to be able to receive multiple inputs from many other neurons and to distribute their outputs to many targets. Thus neurons have taken on a shape illustrated by a generic nerve cell from the mammalian nervous system (Figure 1-2). Like all cells in the body, neurons have a cell body (soma; *plural,* somata) with a nucleus and an especially promi-nent nucleolus, but instead of a rounded or cuboidal cell shape, neurons have cytoplasmic extensions that form an expansive arbor of branching, fingerlike processes called *dendrites.* Most dendrites are decorated with small *spines* that extend like knobs from their surface. The soma and dendrites serve as the parts of a neuron that are specialized for receiving information from other nerve cells. Another single and often quite long process called the *axon* leads away from the cell body and travels for varying distances, eventually branching into numerous axon terminals that end on the dendrites and soma of other nerve cells or onto other targets cells such as muscle fibers or gland cells. All axons are enclosed in membranes of specialized glial cells, and in about half of axons (the larger-diameter ones), the glial membranes make several tight spiral wrappings around segments of the axons, forming a myelin sheath. Thus the

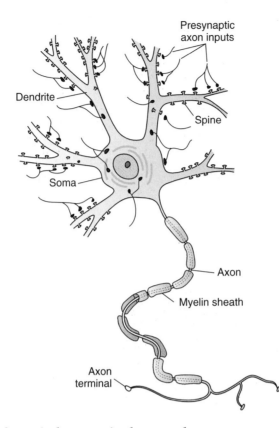

Presynaptic
axon inputs

Dendrite

Spine

Soma

Axon

Myelin sheath

Axon
terminal

Figure 1-2 ■ Drawing of a typical neuron in the central nervous system. Note that the soma (cell body) contains a large nucleus with prominent nucleolus and also contains a Golgi apparatus and numerous stacks of rough endoplasmic reticulum (called *Nissl substance*), which represent the metabolic machinery for synthesizing new membrane and proteins. Most distinctive, however, are the cytoplasmic extensions from the soma. These include multiple dendrites, which often have small spines protruding from them. The full extent of the dendritic tree is not illustrated here but may extend over distances 10 to 100 times the diameter of the soma. Also coming off the soma is a long thin process, the axon, that may travel for long distances, eventually dividing into small terminals, rather bulblike, that end as a presynaptic ending onto the dendrites or soma of other neurons. Many axons are wrapped in a myelin sheath formed by glial cells (oligodendroglia in the central nervous system, Schwann cells in the peripheral nervous system). A few presynaptic axon endings are shown terminating on dendritic spines or on dendrite or soma surface membrane of this neuron. These inputs produce small synaptic potentials that are integrated by the neural membrane and can trigger an action potential near the base of the axon that will propagate down the axon to its terminals, causing release of synaptic transmitter that will influence the membrane potential of the neuron(s) on which this axon terminates.

cell membrane and cytoplasm of neurons is very extensive compared with other cells. The soma typically is composed of less than 5% of the total volume of a neuron. The bulk of the cytoplasm is distributed into the dendrites and axon.

The specialized communication that occurs between an axon terminal and the dendritic or somatic membrane of another neuron is called *synaptic transmission*. The morphological region where the axon terminal abuts against the membrane of a dendrite or cell body is called a *synapse*. The axon terminal is said to be the *pre*synaptic element of a synapse, and the specialized area of dendritic or somatic membrane lying beneath, or adjacent, to the terminal is the *post*synaptic element. An electrical impulse invading the axon terminal leads to the release of a chemical messenger, or *"transmitter,"* from the terminal that then interacts with specialized receptor molecules in the postsynaptic membrane of the receiving cell. The interaction of transmitter and receptor can lead to changes in the electrical activity in the postsynaptic cell and thus influence whether this neuron will also fire an electrical impulse. A significant part of this book deals with the details of synaptic transmission, but for now it is important to appreciate that this capability is the heart of how the nervous system works. In fact, as deduced by Cajal mainly on purely anatomical grounds, nerve cells can be said to have a "dynamic polarity." Their dendrites receive multiple inputs from a host of axon terminals from other neurons. The dendrites and soma integrate all this information and alter the electrical potential of the neuron so as to induce an electrical impulse that travels down the axon of the cell and then causes release of transmitter onto all the targets of this cell. The target cells then integrate this new information with other inputs they receive on their dendrites, and the process of information transfer continues down a chain of nerve cells (Figure 1-3).

■ THE CELL'S LIPOIDAL PLASMA MEMBRANE USES TRANSMEMBRANE PROTEINS TO TRANSPORT MOLECULES AND IONS TO SUPPORT CELLULAR INTEGRITY

Neurons are unique in their ability to sustain and rapidly alter electrical potentials across the cell membranes and to use this capability for remarkable signaling functions. To appreciate the importance of this phenomenon and to understand how it works, the following analogy may be helpful. Imagine a primitive cell as a water-filled balloon; the lipoidal cell membrane is like the rubbery wall of the balloon. Initially, the fluid trapped inside the balloon is the same as the seawater in which the balloon floats. The inside of the balloon may have a nucleus, other organelles, and metabolic machinery. But this cell could not live because its lipoidal membrane, like the balloon wall, is essentially impermeable to polar molecules and salts. (As we know, the plasma membrane is composed of a lipid bilayer, whose major constituents are phospholipids and cholesterol, highly amphipathic compounds whose hydrophobic hydrocarbon tails align to form a sheet that is highly impermeant to water and most polar and charged molecules and ions.) The water and waste products derived from metabolic processes could not escape the cell, and nutritive molecules, like carbohydrates and amino acids, could not cross into the cell. Thus, while the membrane is a marvelous corral that retains and binds closely together in functional proximity the elements of the intracellular compartment, it must provide for a *controlled* exchange of molecules in and out across it. To have the specificity and selectivity necessary for regulation of transmembrane movement of molecules, large protein molecules evolved that were inserted into the lipid matrix of the membrane. These enzyme like proteins serve as transporters or pumps, which, sometimes with the expenditure of energy, readily facilitate the movement of many organic molecules across the otherwise

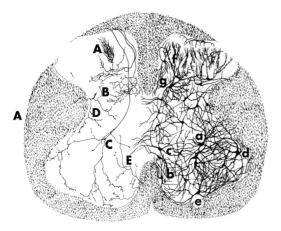

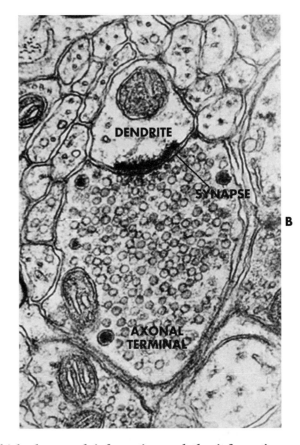

Figure 1-3 ■ Axons have specific targets to which they send information and the information transfer occurs through a synapse. A, Cross-section of kitten spinal cord shows *(left)* the distribution of various types of axons *(A to E)* into different regions of the cord and *(right)* representative neurons *(a to g)* that reside in the spinal cord. Note how the shapes of axon terminals on the *left* would superimpose on specific neurons or dendritic arbors on the right. Even more obvious ordered arrays of axons and dendritic trees can be found in the layers of cerebral and cerebellar cortex. B, Electron micrograph of a typical synapse in the mammalian central nervous system, showing an axon terminal filled with clear round vesicles containing synaptic transmitter. The terminal is making a synaptic contact with a dendrite. (A from Scheibel ME, Scheibel AB: A structural analysis of spinal interneurons and Renshaw cells. In Brazier MAB, ed: *The interneuron*, Los Angeles, 1969, University of California Press, p. 169; B courtesy Richard E. Coggeshall, University of Texas Medical Branch, Galveston, Texas.)

impermeant membrane. Other membrane proteins evolved that allowed facilitated movement of water across the membrane as well.

The metabolic processes of living cells, with the resultant movement of water and organic molecules through the membrane, produced disturbances in osmotic balance that required compensation by shifting dissolved inorganic cations and anions into or out of the cell. In parallel, many such ions were also functioning as important cofactors or regulators of intracellular biochemical events. Thus, in addition to evolving special integral membrane proteins for transporting water and organic molecules, membranes provided pumps that selectively transported a variety of inorganic salts across the membrane. Eventually, these pumps moved enough ions selectively either into or out of the cell that the concentrations of many of the most abundant ions in the extracellular fluid, such as sodium, potassium, chloride and calcium, were markedly different inside the cell. The concentrations of sodium, chloride, and free calcium ions inside of cells, for example, are much lower than the concentrations outside the cell, while the intracellular concentration of potassium is much greater than that outside.

Thus, over a billion years of evolution, all living cells developed large numbers of kinds of integral membrane proteins that regulate the active movements of molecules and solutes through the membrane. These pumps and transporters move otherwise impermeable water, organic molecules, and salts through the membrane and establish a steady-state condition that maintains the living cell. The chemical makeup of the inside of cells, including concentrations of ions, is obviously very different from the outside composition, but osmotic balance is continuously maintained and the integrity of the cytoplasm is protected by the membrane and its array of proteins. It is as if our original balloon were festooned with thousands of elaborate proteins that span its wall and provide selective channels for water flow and carriers for moving molecules and ions across itself.

■ UNEQUAL DISTRIBUTION OF ION CONCENTRATIONS CAN LEAD TO TRANSMEMBRANE POTENTIALS

An unequal distribution of ion concentrations inside and outside a cell can lead to the production of a transmembrane electrical potential difference if the ion can penetrate the membrane. All living cells, including neurons, have established different ion concentrations on either side of their membrane, but there need not be any bioelectricity involved. However, these natural processes set the stage for generation of electrical potentials if cells could evolve a way to take advantage of it.

Recall that cells have pumps and transporters in their membranes, which have caused a redistribution of certain dissolved ions between the inside and outside of cells, mainly in response to metabolic events, proton (H^+) production, and osmotic shifts caused by water movements. Regardless of why it occurred, cells have pumped sodium out of the cytoplasm and pumped potassium ions into the cytoplasm so that the intracellular sodium concentration is about ten times less than that in the extracellular fluid, and the intracellular potassium concentration is about twenty times greater than that outside the cell. This process by itself does not create electrical potentials because whatever the species of cation inside or outside the cell, all the positive cationic charges are balanced, or neutralized, by readily available negative anionic charges such as those on chloride ions outside the cell or on negatively charged molecules inside the cell. (Such intracellular negatively charged molecules include the phospholipid phosphatidylserine in the cytoplasmic side of the lipid bilayer of the membrane and a host of organic compounds with carboxylate, sulfate, and phosphate groups carrying a net negative charge at normal cytoplasmic pH.) So, where does the electrical potential of so-called excitable cells come from? How does an unequal distribution of ions across a membrane lead to the creation of electrical potentials?

The answer is elegant and simple and based on basic principles of thermodynamics. It is, however, one of the most profound accomplishments in biology that cells developed a means to exploit these simple principles. We owe our understanding of these processes to the German physical chemist, Walter H. Nernst. About 100 years ago, Nernst quantitatively demonstrated that if a charged ion, such as potassium (K^+) ions in potassium chloride (KCl), was at two different concentrations on either side of a membrane that was exclusively permeable to that ion, then a small net flow of K^+ ions would move across the membrane, carrying a small but significant positive charge. The concentration gradient alone would force some K^+ ions from the side of higher concentration to the side of lower concentration. As a net flow of K^+ ions occurred, they would carry their charge to the side of the membrane with the lower concentration, creating a net positive charge on that side of the membrane and leaving behind a small net negative charge carried on impermeable anions (chloride [Cl^-] ions in this case) left behind by the net movement of potassium. One side of the membrane would begin to accumulate a net positive potential relative to the other side, but this positive potential would also repel the K^+ ions that were moving toward it (or, equivalently, the K^+ ions would be attracted to the net negativity on the opposite side of the membrane generated by the chloride ions left behind). Eventually, the movement of K^+ ions would be equal in the two directions across the membrane; the ions forced across by the concentration gradient would be balanced by those that were moved in the opposite direction by the electrical field that had been established by the original movement down the concentration gradient. In other words, an equilibrium is reached so that there is no net movement of K^+ ions across the membrane: the two forces acting on the K^+ ions, concentration gradient and electrical gradient (or potential difference), are exactly equal and opposite. The magnitude of the electrical potential established (E) by the movement of K^+ ions is directly proportional to the concentration difference, and Nernst provided an equation that calculated the

size of the potential that would be produced when an ion reaches equilibrium in its flux to the two forces of concentration gradient and electrical field for any concentration difference. When this so-called *equilibrium potential* (E) is achieved, the magnitude of the electrical gradient is equal and opposite to the concentration gradient for that ion across the membrane. The Nernst equation for the equilibrium potential follows:

$$E_{ion} = (RT/FZ)\ln(C^a_{ion}/C^b_{ion})$$

where C^a_{ion} = ion concentration on side "a" of a membrane selectively permeable to the ion, and C^b_{ion} = ion concentration on the opposite side ("b") of the membrane.

This equation is examined in more detail in Chapter 2, but for now we can note that an electrical potential (E) can be generated across a membrane selectively permeable to a particular ion, and the size of the potential can be calculated from constants (that convert moles of ions to electrical charge) multiplied by the logarithm of the concentration ratio of the ion on the two sides of the cell membrane. Note, however, that the ion movements and equilibrium states can be created in entirely passive systems; no energy is required to create these potentials. All that is needed is a concentration difference and a barrier that is permeable to only one of the ions.

This physical-chemical process is directly applicable to living cells. After equilibrium is reached, the cell's potential will be the same as that of the Nernst potential for the permeable ion and no net movement of the ion across the membrane can then occur. All that is required to create an electrical potential across a living membrane is for an ion to be unequally distributed across a membrane and, most importantly, for the membrane to be permeable to the ion.

The universal, transporter-protein–festooned, balloonlike cell described earlier has already accomplished part of what is needed to create electrical potentials. These cells have established, through their pumps, unequal distributions of ions across their membranes. But, since such cells have no way for ions to move passively through their lipid membrane, they cannot establish electrical potentials by any "Nernstian" mechanism. In other words, such cells are impermeant to ions. It can be said that such cells have "theoretical" or "possible" electrical potentials that *could* be established for any ion unequally distributed across the membrane. A Nernst potential can be calculated for Na^+, K^+, Cl^-, Ca^{++}, Mg^+, or any other ion. If the cell could be made exclusively permeable to that ion, so that its concentration gradient would induce a small net transfer of the ion across the membrane and thus set up a charge difference, we could have a potential. But until or unless a mechanism is developed for these membranes to become permeable to ions, the theoretical Nernst equilibrium for any ion cannot be realized.

■ EXCITABLE CELLS HAVE INTEGRAL MEMBRANE PROTEINS THAT PERMIT ION-PERMEATION CHANNELS

It is one of the stunning achievements in all of nature that biological membranes evolved a mechanism for permitting ion permeation. This was accomplished by creating new classes of proteins that insert into the hydrophobic lipid membrane and, by their folding and charge distribution, create hydrophilic pores, or channels, through which ions can freely flow across the membrane. Depending on properties of their amino acid sequence and higher order structural arrangements, different ion-channel proteins are highly selective for different species of ions. There are "sodium channels," "potassium channels," "calcium channels," and many others, some with differing degrees of selectivity.

Thus cells overcame the limitations of ion impermeability. Sodium ions, already ten times more concentrated outside of cells than inside, could now move easily into the cell. The Nernst equation predicts that this concentration gradient would force enough positive sodium ions into the cell that an intracellular potential of around +55 millivolts (mV) would be created. Likewise, the high intracellular potassium ion concentration would push K^+ out of the cell through their membrane channels until −75 mV of internal charge were left behind. Indeed, if all the unequally distributed ions could move freely through the available ion channels, that is, if permeability were unrestricted, all the ions would move across the membrane until they were of equal concentration inside and outside the cell, all the different potentials would cancel one another out, and the system would run down and be useless.

■ OPENING OR CLOSING ("GATING") OF CHANNELS CHANGES MEMBRANE PERMEABILITY AND THUS MEMBRANE POTENTIAL

Cells had to develop a means of regulating their permeability to ions. Even though ion channels were now present, they had to be "gated," that is, opened or closed, selectively so that functionally useful electrical potentials or changes in potentials could be produced. If only potassium channels were opened, then only potassium would move across the membrane. As this occurred, a membrane potential would develop that, if allowed to proceed to equilibrium, would be the same as the potential predicted by the Nernst equation for a 20:1 concentration difference in potassium ions (i.e., cell would develop an internal potential of −75 mV). Similarly, if only sodium channels were opened, this would result in a potential inside the cell of +55 mV. The membrane potential will simply move toward the equilibrium (Nernst) potential for whatever ion the cell is permeable to. Thus *permeability can control the voltage of the cell*. If a cell is permeable to more than one ion, the membrane potential will move to some weighted average of the equilibrium potentials that is proportional to the amount of permeability to each ion. The "Goldman equation," which is examined later, allows one to calculate accurately the membrane potential by taking into account the concentration ratios for the ions and the relative permeability of the membrane to each of the ions.

Excitable cells evolved three major ways of gating their ion channels. All gating is accomplished due to special structural properties of the channel proteins or other molecules closely associated with them. Most channels are closed during the resting state of a cell. Some of these channels are *gated by voltage*, that is, the ion channel protein is sensitive to the transmembrane potential itself and the channel may open if the cell is depolarized (made less negative inside). Certain voltage-gated channels selective for sodium, potassium, or calcium play a crucial role in the production of action potentials and release of synaptic transmitters.

Other families of ion channels are gated by chemical messengers (synaptic transmitters and hormones) and are classified as *ligand-gated channels*. Most are selective for potassium or for both sodium and potassium ions (these are commonly designated *cationic channels*); some are selective for chloride. These play a crucial role in neuron-neuron communication at the synaptic junction. Most ligand-gated channels are closed in the absence of a specific chemical transmitter and are opened transiently in its presence, but some ligand-gated channels are normally open and are closed by their specific ligand.

A third class of gated channel is found particularly in certain sensory neuron endings. These channels are sensitive to mechanical stimuli, such as pressure or physical deformation. These *mechanosensitive channels* open in sensory receptors when appropriately stimulated by some mechanical force and tend to be mainly selective for cations.

One unique class of ion channel is open at all times and apparently insensitive to voltage, chemical ligands, or physical changes in the membrane. These are purely passive (i.e., un-gated) channels, mostly selective for potassium ions, and they account for the resting membrane potential of the neuron and contribute significantly to the passive, "electrotonic" properties of nerve cells.

■ THE CELL MEMBRANE IMPOSES CERTAIN "ELECTROTONIC" RESTRICTIONS ON THE WAYS IN WHICH EXCITABLE CELLS HANDLE POTENTIAL CHANGES

These passive, electrotonic (also referred to as "cable" or "local") properties of membranes are important and are briefly discussed here. These are, in fact, properties common to all living cells and derive from the fact that lipid membranes are extremely poor conductors of electricity. In electrical terms, the membrane behaves like a resistor and capacitor arranged in parallel, a so-called R-C circuit. The charge-storing capacitance is represented by the hydrophobic lipid portion of the membrane that has charged ions aligned on its polar surface, and the resistance is represented (mainly) by the open potassium channels at rest. The functional outcome of this arrangement is that any relatively small change in potential induced in the membrane (as by synaptic transmitters) occurs relatively slowly, dissipates exponentially in time and over the space of the membrane from its point of initiation, is graded in size proportionate to the inducing event, and can be summed with other small changes occurring in near time and space proximity on the membrane. These innate characteristics of the membrane permit the integrative properties of neurons but also limit the speed and distance over which small signals can be conducted. Cell size, geometry, and resting conductance all influence these properties. Convenient universal indices of the functional meaning of these properties are the time constant (τ) and length (or space) constant (λ) of any cell, which are measures of the time or distance, respectively, a small passive electrotonic potential will take to dissipate to 1/e (~$\frac{1}{3}$ or 37%) of its original size. Several factors, such as axon and dendrite diameter and the myelin sheath, have profound effects on the electrotonic properties of neurons and thus alter the electrical behavior of nerve cells, particularly their ability to summate synaptic potentials and conduct action potentials. Teleologically, the creation of voltage-gated ion channels and the action potential was a means of overcoming the limitations of the passive, RC-like membrane and permitting the possibility of discrete and long-distance signaling; nevertheless, even action potential propagation depends on these electrotonic properties of neurons.

■ NEURONS EXECUTE THEIR FUNCTIONS BY ALTERING THEIR PERMEABILITY TO VARIOUS IONS FOR VARYING TIMES

Using a typical neuron as a model, we see that we have a cell with normal metabolic machinery and a host of transporters, carriers, and pumps that use energy to maintain a steady osmotic balance and a constant ion concentration across the membrane. Ion pumps, such as the Na^+-K^+ ATPase molecule, are especially prominent in neurons and maintain a constant ion concentration inside the cell. Because the extracellular ion concentration is also constant under physiological conditions, we can see that *the Nernst (equilibrium) potential for each ion is also constant*, depending solely on the ion-concentration ratio on the two sides of the membrane. Nerve cells also have an abundant number and variety of ion channels in their membrane. Most of these are gated, either by voltage or ligands, but are closed in the resting state. The large number of unique, non-gated potassium channels open at rest leads to a high resting potassium permeability

and thus a negative *resting potential* near the Nernstian (equilibrium) potential for potassium. If any of the gated channels for other ions could be opened, the cell's permeability for these ions would increase and the membrane potential would move away from its resting level and toward the equilibrium potential for whatever ion was made more permeable.

Nerve cells, in fact, work exactly this way. They literally sit and wait at their resting potential for some event that will open gated channels, alter their permeability, and thus change their potential. The most common way for this to occur is for another neuron to release a transmitter substance onto this neuron (most nerve cells receive hundreds or thousands of synaptic inputs from other cells). The transmitter interacts briefly with a specific ligand-gated channel, opening the channel and allowing the flow of ions down their electrochemical gradient. If the particular channel opened by the transmitter were highly selective for sodium ions, for example, sodium ions would rush into the cell, following Nernstian rules, and the membrane potential would become more positive, trying to move toward the equilibrium potential for Na^+. Ligand-gated channel openings are very short lived, however, usually lasting only several milliseconds, and then the channel closes again. Only enough sodium ions can enter the cell through the briefly opened sodium channels to cause a relatively small potential change (few millivolts).

■ CHANNELS ARE INSERTED INTO MEMBRANES AT FUNCTIONALLY CRITICAL MORPHOLOGICAL LOCATIONS

Neurons have many millions of channels in their membrane, with each channel inserted at discrete, specified locations to be in morphological and functional registry with the complex functional anatomy of nerve cells. Specific ligand-gated channels are found immediately juxtaposed beneath the synaptic terminals from other neurons. Non-gated potassium channels responsible for the resting potential are rather uniformly distributed over all parts of the neuron. Mechanosensitive channels are present only in the peripheral axon terminals of sensory neurons. Voltage-gated channels are also distributed in special locations on the neuron, being particularly densely associated with the axon and related parts of the neuron.

■ VOLTAGE-GATED CHANNELS UNDERLIE THE PRODUCTION OF ACTION POTENTIALS

Voltage-gated channels are the most remarkable of the gated channels. There are sets of these channels selective for Na^+, K^+, and for Ca^{++}. In general, these channels are closed at the resting potential, but depolarization of the membrane away from rest toward zero potential causes the channels to open. The sensitivity and response of various voltage-gated channel proteins to depolarization is different. Some channels open sooner or faster than others, but the general rule is that with greater depolarization, more channels are opened and they open faster. Most voltage-gated channels selective for either Na^+ or Ca^{++} ions are also actively *closed* by depolarization, but this process, called *inactivation*, occurs with a brief delay after the depolarization-induced opening of the channel.

It is the voltage-gated channels that are responsible for the generation of the action potential in excitable cells. An action potential is a brief, stereotyped change in membrane potential during which the potential moves from its negative resting value near the equilibrium potential for potassium ions (E_K) in the depolarizing direction beyond zero almost to the sodium equilibrium potential (E_{Na}) and then rapidly repolarizes to its resting potential again. Lasting only a few milliseconds, the action potential comprises an inward rush of sodium ions followed by an outward flow of potassium ions. This sequence of events occurs when a neuron is depolarized enough to open voltage-gated sodium channels. When these channels begin to open, sodium flows inward along its electrochemical gradient and the membrane potential is further depolarized, opening more sodium channels. This process continues until the membrane potential is close to E_{Na}. After this much depolarization has occurred and a millisecond or so of time has elapsed, then two other events take place. First, the sodium inactivation process is turned on and the sodium channels are closed. Second, at about the same time as inactivation is occurring, the depolarization has now opened voltage-gated potassium channels (their voltage sensitivity and opening kinetics are different from those for voltage-gated sodium channels). With the opening of these potassium channels the electrochemical gradient pushes potassium ions out of the cell. Efflux of potassium ions brings the membrane potential back to E_K during this period of high potassium permeability.

■ VOLTAGE CLAMPING IS A POWERFUL TECHNIQUE FOR MEASURING CHANNEL ACTIVITY

The first complete quantitative analysis of the relationships between voltage, permeability, and ionic currents in an excitable cell was made by the British electrophysiologists, Alan Hodgkin and Andrew Huxley, in the early 1950s. They pioneered a technique called the *voltage clamp*, whereby a cell's membrane potential could be rapidly moved to and held at any potential by feedback circuits. They demonstrated the dependence of sodium and potassium permeabilities on membrane potential by measuring transmembrane ion current flows at different holding potentials. Their work provided the first complete demonstration of the manner in which a nerve membrane could produce an action potential by regulating the gating of voltage-sensitive "pores" that were selective for sodium and potassium ions. Since that time, the theoretical "pores" have been identified as molecular channels, and the voltage-clamp technique has been refined and used for measuring the properties and responses of a host of different types of channels.

■ SYNAPTIC POTENTIALS ARE THE SITE OF NERVE CELL INTER-COMMUNICATION AND TYPICALLY UNDERLIE THE PRODUCTION OF ACTION POTENTIALS

Where in normal nerve cells does the depolarization come from that leads to the activation of voltage-sensitive channels and the subsequent action potential? In neurons of the central nervous system the depolarization mainly arises from incoming excitatory postsynaptic potentials. Transmitter released onto a neuron will briefly open ligand-gated channels that permit a small net inward movement of positive charge. The brief inrush of positive ions will cause a small depolarization. A single synaptic response may cause so small a depolarization as to only affect a few nearby voltage-gated sodium channels. But the influence of passive, electrotonic properties of neurons is clear: if more depolarizing synaptic potentials occurred soon enough in time and near enough on the membrane, these could all summate and spread farther before dissipating and thus affect more voltage-sensitive channels. It is when enough numbers of excitatory synaptic potentials summate to reach a great enough depolarization to turn on a threshold number of voltage-gated sodium channels that the irrevocable positive-feedback action-potential sequence is triggered.

Cell morphology and discrete localization of various types of ion channels underlie the ability of neurons to communicate. Neurons receive many synaptic inputs onto their cell bodies and extensive dendritic trees. Each neuron uses its axon to distribute a message to all the post-synaptic cells to which it is connected. The signaling processes rely fundamentally on the ability of neurons to selectively gate populations of ion channels. Neurons operate from a baseline condition of high K^+ permeability and thus an imposed negative resting potential. The soma-dendritic membrane integrates the swarms of incoming synaptic potentials and modulates the resting potential. Enough synaptic depolarization can open strategically placed voltage-gated sodium channels and trigger an action potential. This electrical impulse then propagates to all the axon terminals and induces transmitter release that produces synaptic potentials in the postsynaptic cells.

■ REFERENCES AND ADDITIONAL READINGS

Aidley DJ: *The physiology of excitable cells*, ed 4, Cambridge, 1998, Cambridge University Press.

Aidley DJ, Stanfield PR: *Ion channels: molecules in action*, Cambridge, 1996, Cambridge University Press.

Alberts B, Bray D, Lewis J, et al: *Molecular biology of the cell*, ed 4, New York, 2001, Garland Publishing.

Carpenter MB, Sutin J: *Human neuroanatomy*, Baltimore, 1983, Williams & Wilkins.

De Robertis EDP: *Histopathology of synapses and neurosecretion*, New York, 1964, Macmillan.

Eccles JC: *The physiology of synapses*, New York, 1964, Academic Press.

Hall ZW (ed): *An introduction to molecular neurobiology*, Sunderland, Mass, 1992, Sinauer Associates.

Hille B: *Ionic channels of excitable membranes*, ed 2, Sunderland, Mass, 1992, Sinauer Associates.

Hodgkin AL: *The conduction of the nervous impulse*, Springfield, Ill, 1964, Charles C Thomas.

Johnston D, Wu SM-S: *Foundations of cellular neurophysiology*, Cambridge, Mass, 1995, MIT Press.

Jones EG: *The structural basis of neurobiology*, New York, 1983, Elsevier.

Kandel ER, Schwartz JH, Jessell TM (eds): *Principles of neural science*, ed 4, New York, 2000, McGraw-Hill.

Katz B: *The release of neural transmitter substances*, Springfield, Ill, 1969, Charles C Thomas.

Matthews GG: *Neurobiology: molecules, cells and systems*, ed 2, Malden, Mass, 2001, Blackwell Science.

Murray RW: *Test your understanding of neurophysiology*, Cambridge, 1983, Cambridge University Press.

Nicholls JG, Martin AR, Wallace BG, et al: *From neuron to brain*, ed 4, Sunderland, Mass, 2001, Sinauer Associates.

Nolte J: *The human brain*, ed 5, St Louis, 2001, Mosby.

Peters A, Palay SL, Webster H deF: *The fine structure of the nervous system: the neurons and supporting cells*, ed 3, New York, 1991, Oxford University Press.

Ramón y Cajal S: *Neuron theory or reticular theory? Objective evidence of the anatomical unity of nerve cells* (1908) (translated by Purkiss MU, Fox CA), Madrid, 1954, Consejo Superior de Investigaciones Científicas Instituto Ramón y Cajal.

Smith CUM: *Elements of molecular neurobiology*, New York, 1989, John Wiley & Sons.

Sperelakis N (ed): *Cell physiology source book*, ed 2, San Diego, 1998, Academic Press.

Zigmond MJ, Bloom FE, Landis SC, et al (eds): *Fundamental neuroscience*, New York, 1999, Academic Press.

CHAPTER 2

The Ionic Basis of the Resting Potential

Concepts

1. Excitable cells have an internal negative resting potential that is 50 to 90 mV in magnitude. This potential comes about because ions are present in different concentrations inside and outside the cell, and the membrane of excitable cells has differing permeabilities for different ions.

2. The membrane is selectively permeable to the potassium ion in the resting state.

3. The Nernst equation can be used to calculate the equilibrium potential for an ion, and this potential is the electrical gradient that is equal and opposite of the concentration gradient for that ion across the membrane. There is no net movement of an ion across the membrane when the cell's potential is at that ion's equilibrium potential.

4. The equilibrium potentials for Na^+, K^+, and Cl^- in a typical mammalian neuron are +55 mV, −75 mV, and −65 mV, respectively. When a cell becomes permeable to a particular ion, that ion will move across the membrane in appropriate response to the combined electrical and concentration gradients.

5. The membrane potential always tends to move toward the equilibrium potential for whichever ion it is most permeable.

6. The "sodium pump" is an energy-requiring Na-K exchange transport system that carries sodium ions out of the cell and brings potassium ions into the cell. This pump normally keeps the concentration gradients of these ions constant.

7. The Goldman equation allows one to calculate accurately the resting membrane potential by taking into account the concentration gradients for the major ions and the relative permeability of the membrane to each ion.

8. Pacemaker potentials are slow, rhythmic depolarizations of the resting potential that occur in certain cells such as heart muscle pacemakers. They allow for regular repetitions of activity by slowly changing the cell's permeability from potassium to sodium ions.

■ WHAT DOES A MEMBRANE POTENTIAL LOOK LIKE?

To record the activity of a single nerve cell, the potential set up across the membrane of the cell has to be recorded by measuring the voltage inside the cell compared with that outside the cell. To measure the potential inside, one can use for an electrode a glass capillary micropipette filled with a concentrated salt solution such as 3 M potassium chloride (KCl) (Figure 2-1). (Such a concentrated salt solution is used to conduct electricity and to be similar in composition to the ions inside the cell. The glass wall of the micropipette serves as an insulator and provides rigidity. Such electrodes are also called *micro-electrodes*, or *sharp electrodes*.) One end of this glass tube is pulled out to a fine point with an opening less than a micron in diameter (small enough to cause minimal damage to the neuron when the cell is impaled but electrically continuous with the cell interior via the tiny opening at the tip). A silver wire is inserted into the back

of this electrode, and then the wire is attached through an amplifier to an oscilloscope. Another wire is placed in the bath surrounding the nerve cell and also connected to the amplifier and the oscilloscope. The oscilloscope displays the *potential difference* between the glass electrode tip and the wire in the bath as recorded by the differential amplifier, which detects the difference in the potential between the outside "ground" wire and the micropipette electrode. When both electrodes are in the extracellular fluid, there is obviously no potential difference between them, and the oscilloscope shows no potential difference (0 millivolts, mV). Now, if the tip of the electrode is carefully inserted into the neuron cell body, i.e., we get the membrane of the cell between our two electrodes, a shift in potential can be suddenly seen. The oscilloscope shows that the inside of the cell is polarized some 60 mV negative to the outside solution. This potential will remain steady as long as the cell is at "rest," and thus is termed the *resting*

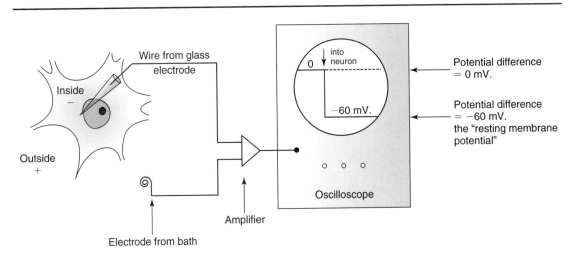

Figure 2-1 ■ A resting membrane potential can be recorded inside a nerve cell. A microelectrode can be used to penetrate a nerve cell, and an amplifier can record the potential difference between the inside of the cell and the surrounding bath. An oscilloscope displays the potential inside the neuron, and this internal potential is typically a negative value of from −50 to −70 mV when the cell is at rest.

membrane potential (RMP), or the *resting potential*. (The exact value of the resting potential varies somewhat from nerve cell to nerve cell but is usually in the range of –50 to –70 mV.)

Two terms are used as convenient definitions to describe displacements from the resting membrane potential. If the internal negative potential is moved toward 0 mV, i.e., made less negative (or the potential difference trace moves upward in our conventional recording system), this is called a *depolarization*. If the membrane potential is made more negative (or in our conventional system, moved downward further from the resting potential), this change is called a *hyperpolarization*.

■ **QUESTIONS**   *(Answers at the end of the chapter)*

1. The inside of excitable cells, such as nerve cells and muscle fibers, has a negative potential in the range of –50 to –90 mV. This steady potential is called the

   _____ .

2. If the resting potential is reduced, i.e., moved toward 0 mV potential, this membrane potential displacement is called a _____ . Conversely, if the resting potential becomes more negative, this is termed a

   _____ .

■ **THE NEURONAL MEMBRANE IS SELECTIVELY PERMEABLE TO IONS**

Nernst Equation and Equilibrium Potentials

The ability of a neuron to maintain the resting potential across its membrane is based on the unequal distribution of ions across the membrane and the selective permeability of the membrane to certain of these ions. Like the membrane of all living cells, the nerve cell membrane has the capability of selectively separating ionic species into different concentrations between the inside and the outside of the cell. Membrane-associated transporter molecules ("pumps") are present that selectively carry ion species either into or out of neurons and maintain constant but different concentrations of most ion species inside and outside the cells (see Table 2-1). Furthermore, having set up these different ionic concentration gradients, membranes allow certain ions to move more readily through the membrane than others, and the membrane is thus said to be selectively, or differentially, permeable. This selective permeability is due to the presence of protein *channels* in the membrane, whose conformational shapes provide hydrophilic pores through which specific ions can traverse the membrane if the channel is open, thus overcoming the hydrophobic barrier established by the lipid bilayer of the membrane. The stereochemical configuration of the channels, the hydrated physical size of ions, and the electrical charges on each are critical factors in determining which ion traverses the membrane. The properties and molecular nature of ionic channels are discussed in more detail later.

It has been demonstrated that if a membrane is exclusively permeable to only one ion, such as potassium, and that ion is distributed across the membrane in unequal concentrations, then an electrical potential will be developed across the membrane. The *Nernst equation* gives the relationship between the magnitude of the electrical potential and the concentration gradient of the ion. Another way of stating the meaning of this very important biological relationship, using an artificial system analogous to a neuron, is as follows:

An ionic species, such as the potassium ions in KCl, may be distributed in unequal concentrations on either side of a membrane selectively permeable to the ion (Figure 2-2, *A*). The concentration difference on the two sides produces a force that causes potassium ions to diffuse across the membrane down their concentration gradi-

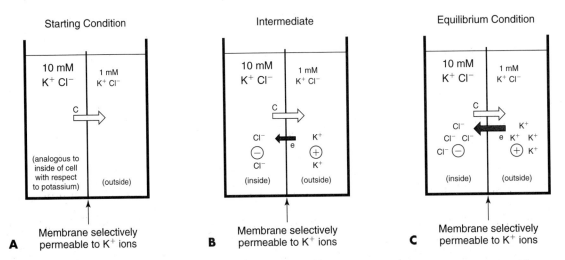

A Membrane selectively permeable to K⁺ ions

B Membrane selectively permeable to K⁺ ions

C Membrane selectively permeable to K⁺ ions

Figure 2-2 ■ Establishment of equilibrium potential. In the starting condition (A) two KCl solutions of different concentration are placed on opposite sides of a membrane that is selectively permeable to K^+ ions and that divides the container in halves. There is a strong concentration gradient *(arrow c)* that will force K^+ ions to the right side of the membrane. This gradient immediately begins to drive K^+ ions through the membrane toward the lower concentration. The movement of K^+ ions down the concentration gradient results in a net shift of positive charges to the right of the membrane and leaves behind a net negativity (Cl^- ions) on the left side. Since K^+ ions are positively charged, they are immediately attracted by this electrical gradient *(arrow e)* to move back to the left (B). K^+ ions will continue to move to the right, however, until enough K^+ ions will have moved rightward that the electrical difference on the two sides will generate an electrical gradient that is exactly equal and opposite in magnitude to the concentration gradient (C). The potential difference that is generated by this movement of K^+ ions imposed by this concentration difference is called the *equilibrium potential*. This term is used because at this potential the movement of K^+ ions through the membrane is in equilibrium; the forces acting on the ions are equal and opposite and an equal number of K^+ ions are moving in both directions through the membrane. At the equilibrium potential there is no net movement of K^+ ions across the membrane in either direction.

---

ent. As the charged K^+ ions move through the membrane, an electrical potential will be developed across it, because a net number of positively charged potassium ions accumulate on one side (that of the lower concentration) and a net number of negatively charged chloride ions are left behind on the other side (Figure 2-2, *B)*. This separation of charge leads to the establishment of an electrical potential across the membrane. As more K^+ ions accumulate on the side of lower K^+ concentration, the magnitude of the

potential increases, and this electrical field will drive K^+ ions back across the membrane, because K^+ ions are repelled by the growing positivity and attracted to the negative environment on the opposite side of the membrane.

This growing potential difference will have a magnitude and direction of force on the charged migrating K^+ ions that are opposite to the force produced on the ions by the concentration gradient. In a brief period of time an equilibrium will be reached, so that for every K^+ ion that moves across the membrane in response to the concentration gradient, there is another K^+ ion that moves across in the opposite direction in response to the electrical gradient (Figure 2-2, C). Thus a *state of equilibrium is attained and there is no net movement of ions across the membrane, although K^+ ions are freely moving across the membrane but at equal rates in both directions.* The electrical potential at which this equilibrium of ion flow is attained is aptly called the *equilibrium potential (E)*. A mathematical expression of the equilibrium potential for a particular ion in a passive system is the Nernst equation:

$$E = RT/FZ \ln (C_1/C_2)$$

where

    E = Equilibrium potential

    R = The gas constant

    T = Absolute temperature

    F = The Faraday constant

    Z = Valence of the ion

    $\ln$ = Natural logarithm

    C_1 = Concentration of ion *outside* the cell

    C_2 = Concentration of ion *inside* the cell

The actual values of the various constants used in the Nernst equation are provided in the answer to text question number 12 on p. 33. What the constants do is convert moles of ions into units of electrical charge. By inserting into the equation the values for these constants, the absolute temperature, the valence of the ion (+ or −), and using 2.3 to change natural logarithms to logarithms with base 10, a simple form of the Nernst equation may be obtained for a monovalent cation in a passive system at 25° C (room temperature), the equation reducing to:

$$E \text{ (in mV)} = 58 \log_{10}(C_1/C_2)$$

Using the example shown in Figure 2-2 and a temperature of 25° C, the equilibrium potential for potassium ions would be:

$$E_K = 58 \log_{10} ([K^+]_o/[K^+]_i)$$

$$E_K = 58 \log_{10} (1 \text{ mM}/10 \text{ mM})$$

$$E_K = 58 \log_{10} (0.1) \ \{\log_{10} \text{ of } 1/10 = -1\}$$

$$E_K = 58 \ (-1)$$

$$E_K = -58 \text{ mV}$$

This means that a potential difference of 58 mV will develop across a membrane selectively permeable to potassium ions simply because of the original concentration gradient on K^+ ions. Several important features of this system should be emphasized.

1. This is an entirely *passive process*; no energy is required to establish the potential. As long as a concentration difference is in place, the energy is already "stored" to make the movement possible. Our own energy was used to prepare the two different ion solutions in our artificial situation in Figure 2-2; the Na^+, K-ATPase pump sets up the concentration difference under normal physiological circumstances in real cells.

2. The number of potassium ions that actually move across the membrane to set up the imbalance of charge is *extremely* small (only a few picomoles, 10^{-12} moles), and thus *the original concentration gradient is not significantly altered*. (This is true because even a small number of charged ions carry significant amounts [coulombs] of electrical charge [see Chapter 3].)

3. Although it may not appear intuitively obvious at first, the side of the membrane with the higher concentration of K^+ ions also has the net negative charge.

4. The Nernst equation is only applicable for systems in which the membrane is highly selectively permeable (really *exclusively permeable*) to only one ion.

5. It does not matter what the negatively charged companion anionic species is that is dissolved with K$^+$ ions, as long as the negatively charged species is not permeant. The solute might be Cl$^-$ ions as in Figure 2-2, but it could be any other negatively charged species such as fixed negative charges on intracellular organic molecules.

6. The ratio of outside ion concentration over inside ion concentration used in the Nernst equation is set by convention to always give the value of the *intracellular potential*. Thus the potential of –58 mV refers to the sign of the potential inside of the cell, and the left side of our artificial experiment in Figure 2-2 was assigned with a higher K$^+$ concentration to be analogous to the intracellular environment.

■ **QUESTIONS** *(Answers at end of chapter)*

3. What is a cation? An anion?

4. What is a selectively permeable membrane?

5. What is the process called whereby an ion moves from a region of high concentration to a region of low concentration?

True or False (Questions 6–8)

6. The force of a concentration gradient may be strong enough to separate two oppositely charged ions across a selectively permeable membrane.

7. An ion in a Nernst equilibrium state cannot move across the membrane.

8. If, in the example shown in Figure 2-2, the membrane had been selectively permeable to Cl$^-$ instead of K$^+$ ions, the final electrical potential established would have been equal and opposite to the one derived for K$^+$ and would be caused by the

transference of a minute number of Cl$^-$ ions from the left to the right of the membrane.

9. Calculate the Nernst (or equilibrium) potential for Cl$^-$ ions in a system such as in Figure 2-2 except that the membrane is selectively permeable to Cl$^-$ ions.

Thus, by knowing the external and internal concentrations of the ion to which a membrane is permeable, one can simply calculate what potential would be generated when the ion moves to reach an equilibrium state across the membrane. The magnitude of the electrical potential is no more than the exact amount of force that is required to counteract the force produced by the concentration gradient. At that equilibrium potential there would be no net movements of the ion across the membrane. A corollary of this situation is that if the membrane's potential were to be displaced by some means, the membrane would "respond" to the change in potential by allowing K$^+$ ions to move across the membrane in response to the voltage change. (Because the membrane is only permeable to K$^+$ ions, they are naturally the only ions that could respond to an imposed change in membrane potential.) So, if a membrane had a membrane potential of –58 mV across it because it was exclusively permeable to K$^+$ ions (Figure 2-3, *A*) and the membrane potential could be artificially changed by depolarizing it by 10 mV to a new potential of –48 mV, this reduction in the negativity of the potential would mean that K$^+$ ions were not being held so strongly on the negative side of the membrane (Figure 2-3, *B*). The reduction in the magnitude of the electrical gradient would permit some K$^+$ ions to cross the membrane in a net outward direction along their concentration gradient. The vectors indicating magnitude and direction of the concentration and electrical forces are no longer

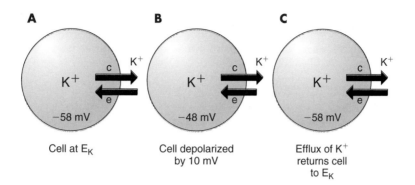

A

B

C

Cell at E_K

Cell depolarized
by 10 mV

Efflux of K^+
returns cell
to E_K

Figure 2-3 ■ **Potassium ions will move across the membrane in response to a change in membrane potential. The drawing in A represents a model nerve cell with an internal potential of –58 mV, the equilibrium potential calculated for a cell with a 1 to 10 ratio of $[K^+]_o/[K^+]_i$. Under these conditions the concentration *(c)* and electrical *(e)* gradients are equal and opposite. In B the cell is depolarized by 10 mV by injecting a brief pulse of positivity into the cell with an electrode. The reduction in internal negativity reduces the electrical gradient holding K^+ ions inside the cell, and there will be a net outward flux of K^+ ions pushed by the constant, and now less opposed, concentration gradient. K^+ ions will leave the cell, making the inside more negative again, and will do so until the electrical gradient of –58 mV is reestablished and the cell is once again at E_K (C).**

equal and opposite; the electrical field vector is decreased (shortened). As the K^+ ions crossed the membrane they would carry away positive charges and the applied voltage change would start to be reduced. The K^+ ions would continue to move away from the less negative internal potential until they had carried away enough positivity to return the membrane potential back in the negative direction to the original equilibrium potential where concentration and electrical gradients are once again balanced (Figure 2-3, *C*). In other words, the ions to which a membrane is permeable are the ones that will respond to imposed changes in transmembrane potential because they are the only ions that can permeate the membrane and the effect of the imposed ion movements will always be to return the membrane potential to the equilibrium potential for the permeable ion.

Studies with many excitable cells have revealed that the resting membrane potential is very near

the potassium equilibrium potential (E_K) calculated from the Nernst equation using the values for intracellular and extracellular potassium concentrations. Table 2-1 shows the concentrations of the main ions found in the cytoplasm and in blood of a typical mammalian nerve cell and in a widely studied model preparation, the giant axon of the squid, which because of its large size and hardiness has proven highly advantageous for neurophysiological experiments.

The Potassium Ion

Many of these early experiments were performed in a real neuron, the squid axon. What should the resting potential be if the cell is actually permeable to K^+ ions? Using the Nernst equation in an experiment at room temperature and knowing that the ratio of the concentration of potassium ions outside $[K^+]_o$ (20 mM) to inside $[K^+]_i$ (400 mM) is 1/20, the potassium equilibrium potential should be:

TABLE 2-1

Concentrations of ions inside and outside representative nerve cells

Ion	Extracellular (mM)	Intracellular (mM)	Ratio: Extracellular/intracellular
Mammalian Neuron			
Na^+	145	15	10/1
K^+	5	125	1/25
Cl^-	125	9	14/1
Ca^{++}	2	10^{-4}	—
A^- (impermeant anions)	—	100	—
Squid Axon			
Na^+	440	50	9/1
K^+	20	400	1/20
Cl^-	560	40	14/1
A^- (impermeant anions)	—	400	—

Values for intracellular concentrations are approximate. The impermeant intracellular anions (A^-) refer to negatively charged organic molecules inside the cell (see Chapter 1). Free Ca^{++} ion concentration within all cells is extremely low, $\leq 10^{-7}$ M. The intracellular and extracellular compartments are each electrically neutral (i.e., all the positive charges are balanced by an equal number of negative charges inside and outside the cell, respectively). The negative and positive charges illustrated here are not equal within a compartment because contributions of numerous other charged species are not included in the table and intracellular values are estimates and differ among cells. It should be noted that, although the absolute concentrations of these various ions differ in the two species, as would be expected on the basis of their respective environments, the ratios of the extracellular and intracellular ion concentrations are comparable.

$$E_K = RT/FZ \ \ln([K^+]_o/[K^+]_i)$$

$$= 58 \log_{10} (1/20)$$

$$= 58 \ (-1.301)$$

$$= -75 \ mV$$

If the cell is exclusively permeable to potassium, then the resting potential measured with a microelectrode should be near E_K, -75mV, and it is ($\sim$ -60mV) (see Figure 2-1). In addition, if $[K^+]_o$ were altered, the resting potential ought to change in a systematic fashion. One would predict that whenever $[K^+]_o$ was changed by a factor of 10 (i.e., one $\log_{10}$ unit), then the resting potential should change by 58 mV. Figure 2-4 shows $[K^+]_o$ in squid blood plotted on a log scale on the abscissa and membrane potential given on the ordinate, plotted in the same way it was recorded, with internal negativity downward. The solid theoretical line is, of course, a straight line plotted from the Nernst equation, and the observed points from our experiment, plotted as the dotted line, fit the predicted values very well, except in the region of low $[K^+]_o$ near the resting potential. Although a membrane potential of -75 mV would be expected if the membrane accurately followed the Nernst equation, the mem-

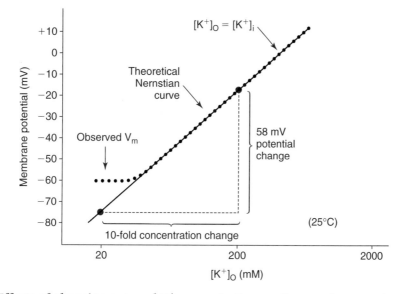

Figure 2-4 ■ **Effects of changing external K$^+$ concentration on the membrane potential of a squid axon. Plotted on the abscissa on a log scale is the external concentration of K$^+$ ions. On the ordinate is plotted membrane potential. At rest, the internal potential (V$_m$) recorded is –60 mV with a normal [K$^+$]$_o$ of 20 mM. When the extracellular [K$^+$] is increased, an ever-decreasing V$_m$ is measured (dotted line). The equilibrium potential predicted by the Nernst equation for varying [K$^+$]$_o$ is plotted as the solid line, with V$_m$ changing 58 mV for every 10-fold change in [K$^+$]$_o$. Except for values of V$_m$ near the resting potential, the experimental points (dotted line) match the theoretical line very well. If the membrane were exclusively, perfectly permeable to K$^+$, V$_m$ should be –75 mV at the normal [K$^+$]$_o$ of 20 mM.**

brane potential is actually –60 mV at normal [K$^+$]$_o$. Otherwise, the agreement between the observed and expected results is excellent. Because the resting membrane potential follows the predicted Nernst equation values for potassium so closely, it can be inferred that *the resting membrane is very permeable to potassium and impermeable or only slightly permeable to other ions.*

How does this distribution of potassium ions in a real cell actually cause an electrical potential? Consider a neuron that is filled with a high concentration of K$^+$, a low concentration of Na$^+$ and Cl$^-$, and a high concentration of internal anions (A$^-$) and assume that the membrane is permeable to potassium ions and impermeable

to sodium, chloride, and the internal anions. If this neuron is put in a bath that contains Na$^+$, Cl$^-$, and very little K$^+$, what will happen to the potassium ions? Clearly, the concentration gradient on potassium is directed outward, because there is 20 times more K$^+$ inside than outside. Accordingly, potassium ions will leave the cell. However, they are not accompanied by the internal anions, which are not free to move across the membrane. What will happen to the distribution of charge across the membrane? As potassium ions move out, they will, because they are positively charged, make the outside solution more positive and the inside fluid more negative. What will be the effect of this electrical potential? It will tend to prevent potassium ions from leaving the cell (the internal negativity will tend to hold K$^+$ ions inside). How long then will potassium continue to leave the neuron down the concentration gradient? Potassium ions will leave the cell until the electrical force that opposes their leaving is exactly equal to the concentration gradient that is trying to make them leave. This situation is exactly analogous to the system described earlier in Figure 2-1 and is no more than a verbal description of the Nernst equation in which E$_K$ represents the electrical force, and (RT/FZ) ln ([K$^+$]$_o$/[K$^+$]$_i$) represents the concentration force converted to electrical terms. When the membrane potential is at the equilibrium potential E$_K$ (i.e., when the electrical force exactly balances the concentration force), then there will be no net movement of potassium current across the membrane. Thus, at the equilibrium potential for an ion, that ion cannot carry any net current through the membrane. On the other hand, whenever the concentration gradient is not exactly balanced by the electrical gradient, potassium will tend to move in or out and act as a current. It can also be said that at the equilibrium potential no work is required to keep the membrane potential steady, and it will stay there unless something happens to push it away from this value.

■ **QUESTIONS**   *(Answers at end of chapter)*

10. What is a famous invertebrate preparation widely used for studies of the properties of excitable membranes? Why is this a popular experimental preparation?

11. Why is the membrane potential zero when the concentrations of potassium inside and outside the cell are equal?

12. Calculate the Nernst potential for potassium in a typical squid axon at 25° C using the concentrations given in Table 2-1.

13. What would happen to the resting membrane potential if the external potassium concentration were increased?

14. If a cell were selectively permeable to K$^+$ ions and sitting at a normal resting potential of –60 mV, what would happen to the potassium ions if you artificially applied a steady depolarizing electrical current to the inside of the cell?

The Sodium Ion

How are the concentration forces and the electrical forces oriented with respect to the sodium ion for a neuron at the resting membrane potential? There are about 10 times more Na$^+$ ions outside than inside the cell, so the concentration gradient is clearly trying to push sodium into the cell. The membrane potential at rest is negative inside, positive outside, so there is an electrical gradient oriented to bring Na$^+$ into the cell as well. The equilibrium potential for sodium computed from the Nernst equation is E$_{Na}$ = 58 log$_{10}$ (440 mM/50 mM), and E$_{Na}$ works out to be about +55 mV. So, if the membrane were to become permeable to sodium, these ions would rush into the cell. Not until the internal potential reached +55 mV would there be a great enough electrical field driving sodium out to match the concentration gradient pushing sodium in. Indeed, the difference between the resting potential (V$_m$, –60 mV) and E$_{Na}$ (+55 mV) is approximately –115 mV (–60 – [+55] = –115), a strong driving electrical force indeed. Why does sodium not enter the cell at the resting membrane potential, and why is the membrane potential not nearer E$_{Na}$? *Because the membrane at rest is almost completely impermeable to sodium.*

There is, however, a very small amount of "resting permeability" to sodium, and this allows a small amount of sodium to cross into the membrane. As sodium leaks into the cell, positive charges are brought inside, tending to depolarize the cell away from E_K. The effect of this will be to reduce the electrical driving force holding potassium in, and K^+ will leak out (see Figure 2-3 and question 14 for an analogous situation). Potassium apparently leaks out at about the same rate that sodium leaks in; in other words, the outward potassium current is equal and opposite to the inward sodium current. Under these conditions, the membrane potential, V_m, could reach a steady state and be constant at some value a little depolarized from E_K, but would not be at equilibrium because of the small but continuous potassium and sodium fluxes. Because some sodium is always leaking in, we can see why our recorded resting potential (see Figure 2-4) was at –60mV instead of –75mV, E_K. The membrane potential remains in this steady state because the leakage rate is low and because there is a *pump* that can actively transport the sodium ions back out of the cell against their electrochemical gradient and bring the potassium ions back in against their concentration gradient, thus maintaining constant intracellular concentrations of these ions.

■ **QUESTIONS**   *(Answers at end of chapter)*

15. Compute the equilibrium potential for sodium in a mammalian neuron. Use the Nernst equation and concentrations given in Table 2-1.

16. If a nerve were placed in a solution containing only 10% of the normal extracellular sodium concentration, what would the sodium equilibrium potential now be? Would the resting membrane potential be altered, and if so, how?

17. If the membrane were to change its permeability state from being selectively permeable to K^+ to being exclusively permeable to Na^+ ions, what would the new

membrane potential be? (Assume an outside/inside concentration ratio for Na^+ of 10.)

18. Would it be appropriate to deduce from the preceding discussion that the real resting membrane is not perfectly selective in its permeability and that the degree to which the cell is permeable to various ions would be reflected in where the membrane potential is relative to the equilibrium potentials for the various ions?

The Sodium Pump

Within the plasma membrane of all cells and in abundance in excitable cells, there is an enzyme-like protein carrier system *(Na⁺, K⁺-ATPase)* that, with the expenditure of metabolic energy (ATP), has the capability of transporting, or "pumping," Na^+ and K^+ ions through the membrane against their respective concentration gradients. This so-called sodium pump is named mainly for its most obvious function of compensating for the inward leak of sodium ions, as discussed previously. It is, in fact, a "coupled pump" (antiport) that *carries potassium into and sodium out of the cell*. In each cycle of activity with the hydrolysis of one ATP molecule, the pump expels three sodium ions and brings in two potassium ions. The pump then may not be electrically neutral in all neurons since it can cause a net transfer of positivity out of the cell. This "electrogenic" effect can directly add increased negativity to the resting potential, but for most cells it accounts for only a few percent of the total resting potential. Thus any possible electrogenic contribution of the sodium pump to the resting membrane potential generally can be ignored. The sodium pump is selectively poisoned by the cardiac glycoside ouabain, is slowed by cooling, and is sensitive to the internal sodium concentration and the external potassium concentration. Increases in either will cause the pumping rate to go up. At this time, the important fact is that all neurons have such pumps that are essential for maintaining the proper internal sodium and potassium concentrations. *The sodium pump is so effective and efficient that it is correct to assume that in normal neurons the sodium pump is able to compensate for ionic leaks and the concentration gradients (and thus the equilibrium potentials) for sodium and potassium ions are fixed and stable.*

■ **QUESTIONS**   *(Answers at end of chapter)*

19. The sodium pump uses the energy source
    _____ to transport
    _____ ions out of the cell
    and _____ ions into the
    cell.

20. What are two factors that could block or slow down the sodium pump? What is an effective means of increasing its rate of activity?

21. Under normal circumstances, what is the most important consequence of sodium pump activity?

The Chloride Ion

What are the driving forces on Cl⁻ at the resting potential? The concentration gradient is tending to push chloride into the cell, and the electrical gradient is trying to push chloride out. (Remember that Cl⁻ is negatively charged and the inside of the neuron is negative.) The chloride equilibrium potential is usually near or a few millivolts more negative than the resting membrane potential in mammalian neurons. Neural and muscle membranes have a small resting permeability to chloride ions, but these ions are said to be "passively" distributed across the membrane. Because of the small resting permeability to chloride ions, they normally move across the membrane in response to shifts in membrane potential. If the membrane potential changes for any reason, chlo-

ride simply moves outward or inward in appropriate response to the electrical forces so that it once again is near equilibrium at the new membrane potential. The behavior of chloride ions is analogous to that of K⁺ as discussed above (see Figure 2-3) in response to changes in potential, although Cl⁻ ions would move in an opposite direction to K⁺ because of their opposite ionic charge. The main thing to remember is that the permeability to chloride does *not* change at rest or during the action potential. A condition is known where chloride permeability does change; this occurs at the inhibitory synapse, a phenomenon that will be discussed in Chapters 6 and 7.

■ **QUESTION**   *(Answers at end of chapter)*

22. Calculate the equilibrium potential for chloride ions given an outside to inside concentration ratio of 14/1 at a temperature of 25° C.

■ **THE GOLDMAN EQUATION HELPS ACCOUNT FOR THE CONTRIBUTIONS OF MULTIPLE IONIC PERMEABILITIES TO THE RESTING MEMBRANE POTENTIAL**

As implied in the preceding discussion, the permeability of the membrane is different for different ions in the resting state. Conversely, the ability of an ion to affect a transmembrane potential depends on the permeability of the membrane to that ion. If a membrane is not permeable to an ion, that ion's presence—no matter what concentration gradient might exist—does not affect the membrane potential. On the other hand, every ionic species has at least a theoretical equilibrium potential, and if the cell were selectively (exclusively) permeable to that ion, the membrane potential would be at that ion's equilibrium (Nernstian) potential. In fact, the membrane potential will approach an ion's equilibrium potential in proportion to the degree that the cell is permeable to the ion. An important concept to keep in mind is that *the membrane potential will always tend to move toward the equilibrium potential for whichever ion(s) it is permeable*. If, as in examples already discussed, the cell were permeable only to potassium, the membrane potential, V_m, would be at E_K (Figure 2-5, *B*). If the cell were permeable only to Na^+, V_m would be at E_{Na} (Figure 2-5, *C*). If the cell were equally permeable to Na^+ and K^+, then it would be reasonable to suppose that V_m would be halfway between E_{Na} and E_K, the average of the two equilibrium potentials being $([+55] + [-75])/2 = -20/2 = -10$ mV, as shown in Figure 2-5, *D*. In the resting state, the ratio of the permeabilities of the squid axon membrane for the ions K^+, Na^+, and Cl^- is about 10.0:0.4:4.5 (i.e., the membrane at rest is over 20 times more permeable to potassium than to sodium and therefore the resting potential is very near E_K). The permeability to Cl^- is also relatively high, and this would tend to hold V_m near E_{Cl}, an equilibrium value near the resting level as well (Figure 2-5). The relatively low sodium permeability, representing the "sodium leak," accounts mainly for the slight depolarizing shift in V_m to –60 mV, away from the pure potassium permeability-based V_m of –75 mV.

An equation has been developed that takes into account that the resting membrane potential is composed of the contribution of gradient forces on different ions with different permeabilities. It expresses the transmembrane potential as a function of the monovalent ion concentrations and the relative permeabilities of the membrane to these ions. This formulation is the Goldman equation:

$$Vm = \frac{RT}{F} \ln \frac{P_K[K^+]_o + P_{Na}[Na^+]_o + P_{Cl}[Cl^-]_i}{P_K[K^+]_i + P_{Na}[Na^+]_i + P_{Cl}[Cl^-]_o}$$

where

VM = Resting membrane potential
P_X = Permeability to ion X

$[X]_o$ = Extracellular concentration of ion X
$[X]_I$ = Intracellular concentration of ion X

NOTE: Ions of differing valence are involved, so the Z term cannot appear in the formula; chloride's contribution to the resting potential (negative valence) is accounted for by placing its internal concentration in the numerator and its outside concentration in the denominator.

Thus, if the concentrations of these ions inside and outside and the permeabilities of the membrane for each one are known, a very accurate determination of the membrane potential can be computed.

The concepts depicted in Figure 2-5 can be converted into a quasi-electrical model of how permeability can influence membrane potential. In Figure 2-6 a kind of electrical circuit has been superimposed over the plasma membrane. The inside and outside of the cell is connected over four parallel pathways that can contribute to membrane currents. These pathways are considered in a more formal way in Chapter 3, but for now it should be appreciated that membranes can accommodate flow of ionic current through specific and independent channels for K^+, Na^+, and Cl^- ions. Each of these respective pathways is shown by a circuit that contains a variable resistor that represents the permeability to the ion and a battery that represents the equilibrium potential for the ion. The circuit tells us that if the cell had a very high permeability to K^+ ions (i.e., the resistance to K^+ ions was very low), then K^+ ions could easily move through the circuit and set a membrane potential equal to E_K. However, if the resistance to Na^+ ions was low (i.e., P_{Na} were high), then sodium current would move through the membrane until the membrane potential were equal to E_{Na}. Obviously, varying the amount of permeability to different ions would lead to a "blend" of ionic currents and a setting of membrane potential that was a balance of the equilibrium potentials propor-

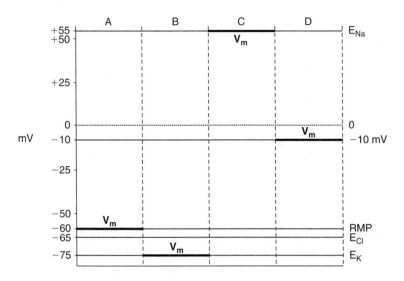

Figure 2-5 ■ The membrane potential moves toward the equilibrium potential for the ion to which it is permeable. The membrane potential, V_m *(heavy line segments),* may be at various levels depending on equilibrium potentials for different ions and the degree to which the membrane is permeable to the ions. The ordinate shows membrane potential in millivolts with the sodium (E_{Na}), potassium (E_K), and chloride (E_{Cl}) equilibrium potentials and resting potential (–60mV) highlighted. Panel *A* shows V_m to be at the normal resting potential. V_m would hyperpolarize to –75mV, E_K, if the cell were exclusively permeable to K^+ ions (panel *B*). If the membrane became exclusively permeable to sodium (panel *C*), V_m would shift to E_{Na} (+55 mV). Normally, nerve membranes have varying degrees of permeability to different ions, and V_m will be somewhere between equilibrium potentials at a level proportional to the permeability to the ions. *D* shows an example of V_m in a cell equally permeable to Na^+ and K^+; the membrane potential is exactly halfway between E_{Na} (+55 mV) and E_K (–75 mV), a value of –10mV.

tional to the resistance of each ion's circuit line.

■ PACEMAKER POTENTIALS

In most excitable cells the membrane potential remains in a stable resting condition at a membrane potential that is determined by a steady-state balance between two or more membrane permeability states. Some nerve cells, smooth muscle, and cardiac cells, however, are known to undergo spontaneous or endogenous fluctuations in their resting potentials and to fire action potentials in a regular or bursting fashion. These

types of cells have a resting potential that oscillates regularly, producing slow continuous depolarizations called *pacemaker potentials.* Instead of maintaining a steady-state resting condition, the cell varies its permeability state over time so that it becomes more permeable to sodium and/or calcium ions and less permeable to potassium ions, and the resting potential drifts in the depolarizing direction. In pacemaker cells of the heart (e.g., those of the sinoatrial node), at the completion of an action potential, the post-spike hyperpolarization turns on a unique, slowly increasing sodium permeability that is accom-

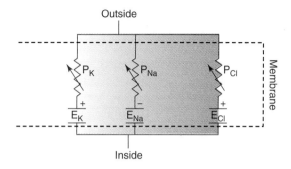

Figure 2-6 ■ **The concept of permeability determining voltage can be illustrated with this simplistic electrical model of the membrane. The model shows three different transmembrane pathways for ions, one each for K^+, Na^+, and Cl^- ions. The permeability of the membrane to each ion is indicated by a variable resistor: high permeability can be thought of as equivalent to a low-resistance pathway. The battery that drives each of the ions is determined by the equilibrium potential for that ion. If the membrane is exclusively permeable to a single ion, then the resistance to that ion's flow will be low and the membrane potential will approach that ion's equilibrium potential. The contribution of each ion's equilibrium potential to the membrane potential will be proportional to the permeability of the membrane to that ion, as discussed for the Goldman equation. A more elaborate and formal representation of the electrical model of the membrane is discussed in Chapter 3.**

panied by a progressive decrease in permeability to potassium ions. The membrane potential is thus less influenced by the hyperpolarizing drive toward E_K and drifts in the depolarizing direction toward the sodium equilibrium potential. The cell's permeability to sodium is, in a relative sense, becoming greater as potassium permeability is decreased. Thus pacemaker cell membrane potentials slowly depolarize until threshold is reached and an action potential, which may involve sodium and calcium ions, ensues; after which the cycle is begun again. It is

not certain how pacemaker cell membranes are able to regulate their permeability in this regularly repeating fashion, but it is known that the phenomenon is a built-in, spontaneous rhythm that does not depend on other input to the cell.

■ **QUESTIONS** *(Answers at end of chapter)*

23. The membrane potential of a cell would drift in the depolarizing direction if _____ permeability were increased, or if _____ permeability were decreased.

24. What are two common characteristics of pacemaker potentials?

Potassium Channels

The results discussed to this point are based on simple thermodynamic principles, and the ionic basis of the resting potential was established on sound theoretical and experimental grounds by mid-century. Although there was solid evidence at a macroscopic level for membranes having selective permeabilities, little was known about the molecular basis for ion permeation. Plus, although it was clear that membranes had some form of "pores" that permitted selected ions to move through them, the nature of these "channels" and how they interacted with the hydrophobic lipid bilayer of cell membranes and regulated ion movements was unknown. In the past few decades, new technologies and new knowledge about biochemistry, structural biology, and molecular biology have revolutionized our understanding of the nature and behavior of ion channels. As outlined in Chapter 1, from the beginning, living membranes were faced with the problem of overcoming the energy barrier of getting charged and polar compounds through the very hydrophobic matrix of the lipid bilayer of phospholipid hydrocarbon tails. Nature's strategy was to build proteins that could be inserted into the bilayer. The basic blueprint for the design of the proteins was to synthesize a relatively large polypeptide molecule that would span across the membrane with parts of the protein exposed to the extracellular environment and parts sticking into the cytoplasm. In the interior of the protein there occurred a series of 20 to 30 amino acids, most with relatively hydrophobic side groups, that, by strong hydrogen bonding among the chain of amino acids and little bonding with water, formed a coil called an *α-helix structure*. This stretch of α-helix could be inserted through the bilayer and held there by weak forces between the hydrophobic side groups of the helix residues and the fatty acid tails of the phospholipids (Figure 2-7, *A*). These are integral membrane proteins, and, although they can move fairly easily laterally in the membrane and come into close association with one another, they cannot flip-flop or tumble over in the membrane. Different proteins have varying numbers of α-helices, so that some have only one and are said to be "single-pass" transmembrane proteins. Many are multi-pass proteins and may have from two to over a dozen transmembrane-spanning α-helices.

Not every amino acid residue in the α-helix is hydrophobic. Some of the amino acids are neutral, a few have slightly polar side groups. Thus two or more α-helix chains have a certain affinity for one another. If a group of α-helices came into close association with their relative hydrophilic residues interacting with one another, one can imagine that a small cylinder, or core, of a relatively hydrophilic nature could be created through this protein-lined space in the midst of a surrounding hydrophobic membrane environment. In essence, this is the basic scaffolding for building a channel through the membrane.

There is good evidence based on molecular biology, genetics, and the structure of channels in the membranes of animals extant today, from prokaryotes to humans, that the most likely original channel created was one for potassium ions. The channel was most likely formed by the association of four nearly identical proteins, each with two membrane-spanning α-helices (Figure 2-7, *B* and *C*). Potassium channels of this general structure can be found in certain bacteria today as well as in mammalian cells, where one such type of channel is an inward rectifier channel for potassium, activated by membrane hyperpolarization. Recent studies with molecular cloning and expression systems, amino acid substitutions (point mutations made by altering nucleotides in the DNA to code for an amino acid different from the naturally occurring one in order to determine whether a particular residue has an important functional or structural role in a channel), and especially crystallization of one of these family members to determine its three-dimensional (quaternary) structure have revealed remarkable insights into the way this channel selects for K^+ ions and facilitates their rapid movement through the channel. Indeed, parts of the helices create a favorable cavity for potassium ions and their waters of hydration to transit much of the membrane width rapidly, and loops of the extracellular domains of the protein and subsets of the helices form an elegantly designed selectivity filter at the extracellular mouth of the channel of exactly the correct dimensions, order and charge to permit only K^+ ions to enter the channel.

Descendants or close relatives of this form of K^+ channel comprise a family of potassium channels found in prokaryotes and all eukaryotes and are believed to represent the molecular structure of the potassium channel responsible for the resting potential. These channels are likely formed by association of an unknown number of subunits, each composed of a single large protein that contains a total of four transmembrane α-helical domains (Figure 2-7, *D*). The four domains represent two repeats of amino acid sequence, each of which is very similar to the single subunit of the older K^+ channel that has two membrane-

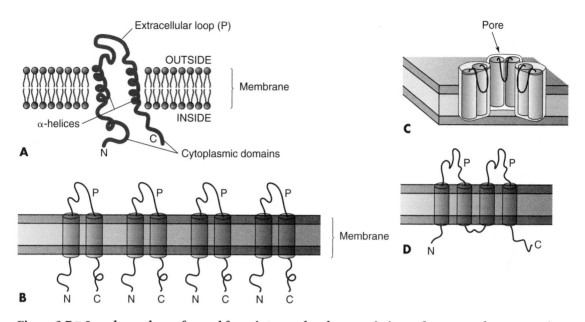

Figure 2-7 ■ Ion channels are formed from inter-molecular associations of transmembrane proteins. All living cells synthesize large proteins that can be inserted into their plasma membranes. Such a transmembrane protein is schematized in A. This protein has two membrane-spanning areas (others may have only one, or may have over 12 such regions) linked by an extracellular loop of protein between the two and with other ends of the protein extending into the cytoplasm. The transmembrane areas are formed by a stretch of 20 to 30 amino acids that form a tight coil called an α-helix. The helix forms strong (but non-covalent) bonds with the hydrocarbon tails of the phospholipids comprising the lipid bilayer. B represents four roughly identical proteins, each a transmembrane protein with two α-helices now represented as a cylinder. In some cells these four proteins can interact in the membrane to form a channel that is selective for potassium ions (C). In this rendition, only three subunits are shown in order to appreciate the topology of the pore. It is believed that the potassium channel that is open in the resting membrane of many excitable cells (D) is a close relative of the protein ensemble in B but is actually comprised of two or more subunits, each of which is a single protein having four transmembrane domains that are homologous to two of the four double-helix structures in B. Again, in an assembly analogous to that depicted in C, a selective and fast through-put channel for K^+ ions is believed to be formed by the quaternary structure of an ensemble of multiple numbers of these protein subunits to serve as the resting membrane K^+ channels.

---

spanning α-helices (Figure 2-7, *B*). More distantly related potassium-selective channels exist, some gated by voltage, others by chemical transmitters or modulators. These channels are explored in later chapters.

■ **SUMMARY**

In the membranes of excitable cells there are many of the "resting" K^+ channels per square micron of membrane surface. The channels are open all the time and are not gated. They permit the ready movement of K^+ ions, hundreds of thousands of ions per second, in either direction through the membrane, the ions flowing immediately in response to any perturbation in transmembrane electrical gradient that acts on them. They are clearly the molecular substrate for the high resting permeability of excitable cells to potassium.

■ POST-TEST

1. What is responsible for a neuron's ability to maintain a steady state constant internal sodium concentration?

2. (a) Explain briefly the meaning of the Goldman equation
   (b) Using the following values, compute the ratio P_{Na}/P_K for a cell at rest:

V_m (resting potential) =	–65 mV
Temperature =	25° C
$[K^+]_o$ =	20 mM
$[Na^+]_o$ =	450 mM
$[Cl^-]_o$ =	560 mM
$[K^+]_i$ =	400 mM
$[Na^+]_i$ =	50 mM
$[Cl^-]_i$ =	40 mM
P_K =	0.23 mmho/cm^2
P_{Cl} =	0.26 mmho/cm^2

   (c) Would this ratio ever change during the existence of a neuron?

3. What would happen to the resting potential if a small amount of negative current were artificially injected into the cell? How would the movement of K^+ ions then counteract this effect? Why would we expect K^+ ions to do so?

4. The membrane potential will approach the _____ for the ion to which it is _____ .

5. What is the ratio of resting permeabilities for K^+, Na^+, and Cl^- in squid axon membrane?

6. What are the meanings for the following terms expressing aspects of membrane voltage or potential: V_m, resting membrane potential (RMP), and E_{ion}?

■ REFERENCES AND ADDITIONAL READINGS

Baker PF, Hodgkin AL, Shaw TI: The effects of changes in internal ionic concentrations on the electrical properties of perfused giant axons, *J Physiol* (London) 164:355-374, 1962.

DeFrancesco D: Pacemaker mechanisms in cardiac tissue, *Annu Rev Physiol* 55:455-472, 1993.

Doyle DA, Cabral JM, Pfuetzner RA, et al: The structure of the potassium channel: molecular basis of K$^+$ conduction and selectivity, *Science* 280:69-77, 1998.

Goldman DE: Potential, impedance, and rectification in membranes, *J Gen Physiol* 27:37-60, 1943.

Hodgkin AL, Katz B: The effect of sodium ions on the electrical activity of the giant axon of the squid, *J Physiol* (London) 108:7-77, 1949.

Hodgkin AL, Keynes RD: Active transport of cations in giant axons from *Sepia* and *Loligo, J Physiol* (London) 128: 28-60, 1955.

Horisberger J-D, Lemas V, Kraehenbühl J-P, et al: Structure-function relationship of Na, K-ATPase, *Annu Rev Physiol* 53:565-584, 1991.

Nernst W: On the kinetics of substances in solution. Translated from *Z Phys Chem* 2: 613-622, 1888. In Kepner GR (ed): *Cell membrane permeability and transport*, Stroudsburg, Penn, 1979, Dowden, Hutchinson & Ross, pp. 174-183.

Thomas RC: Electrogenic sodium pump in nerve and muscle cells, *Physiol Rev* 53:563-594, 1972.

■ ANSWERS
Text Questions

1. Resting potential.

2. Depolarization; hyperpolarization.

3. A cation is a *positively* charged ion (like Na$^+$ or K$^+$); an anion is a *negatively* charged ion (like Cl$^-$).

4. A membrane that is exclusively, or differentially, more permeable to certain ions than to others.

5. Diffusion (down a concentration gradient).

6. True.

7. False. The ion moves back and forth through the membrane under the influence of the concentration and electrical gradients, but there is *no net movement*.

8. True.

9. $E_{Cl} = RT/FZ \ln ([Cl^-]_o/[Cl^-]_i)$.
   Since the valence of Cl^- is -1, at 25° C, $[(RT/FZ) \ln]$ converts to $-58 \log_{10}$; thus
   $E_{Cl} = -58 \log_{10} (1/10)$.
   $E_{Cl} = -58 (-1)$
   $E_{Cl} = +58$ mV

This means that as chloride ions moved from left to right in Figure 2-2, they would leave behind a positive potential on the left side of the membrane. Cl^- ions would continue to move down their concentration gradient to the right until the positivity on the left (or the accumulating negativity on the right) was enough to counteract the concentration gradient. (Important note: this distribution of Cl^- ions is *opposite* to that of a normal cell, which has little intracellular Cl^- and a large extracellular Cl^- concentration.)

10. The *giant axon of the squid* is a very advantageous preparation for the study of excitable membranes because it is large (sometimes a millimeter in diameter) and a stable, hardy preparation. (This is also a very accessible preparation that is easy to dissect and work with.) It is large enough to allow multiple electrode penetrations and to provide adequate amounts of cytoplasm to make direct measurements of ion concentrations. The inside of the axon can be perfused with solutions of different concentrations of ions. Nobel Prize–winning research has been done with the squid axon, and this exceptional model system is discussed in Chapter 3.)

11. When $[K^+]_o = [K^+]_i$, the Nernst equation would be:
    $E_K = 58 \log_{10} [K^+]_o /[K^+]_i$
    $= 58 \log_{10} (1)$; the $\log_{10}$ of $1 = 0$
    $E_K = 0$ mV.

Find this point on the graph in Figure 2-4.

12. As an example, a complete calculation of the Nernst equation for potassium is given:
    Nernst equation: $E = RT/ FZ \ln (C_1/C_2)$

    where
    E = Equilibrium potential in volts
    R = Gas constant, 8.31 joules/g mole/deg [units of a joule are volts × coulombs]
    T = Absolute temperature (273 degrees Kelvin + degrees C)
    F = Faraday, 96,500 coulombs/g mole
    Z = Valance of ion, no units
    ln = Natural logarithm; may be converted to $\log_{10}$ by multiplying by 2.3
    C_1 = External concentration of ion
    C_2 = Internal concentration of ion

    For potassium:
    $E_K = RT/FZ \ln ([K^+]_o/[K^+]_i$, for temperature of 25° C
    $= \{[8.31$ volts × coulombs/g mole/deg $(273 + 25$ degrees$)]/[96,500$ coulombs/g mole $(+1)]\} \times (2.3) \log_{10}(20/400)$
    $= [0.059$ volts$] \log_{10} (0.05)$
    $= 0.059$ volts (-1.301)
    $E_K = -0.076$ volts, or
    $E_K = -76$ millivolts (mV)

13. The cell would be depolarized; note that the ratio of outside to inside potassium concentrations would be decreased, making the results of the Nernst calculation less negative.

14. When the cell was depolarized by l0 mV so that the resting potential was shifted from –60 to –50 mV, the electrical gradient tending to attract K^+ ions into the cell would be reduced. (Remember that normally the concentration gradient had pushed out enough potassium to set up a residual –60 mV attractive force inside). With less negativity inside to attract or hold the potassium ions inward, the force of the concentration gradient would allow a net flow of K^+ ions *outward* (i.e., the outward concentration gradient would no longer be balanced by an equal and opposite electrical gradient). For an equivalent situation, note that the "e" arrow in Figure 2-3, *B,* is "shorter" than the "c" arrow. Thus the resting cell would respond to an imposed depolarization by allowing a passive outward flow of K^+ ions. As long as an imposed depolarization continues due to positivity being added to the inside of a cell by an electrode, K^+ ions will leave the cell at the same rate positivity is being injected. When the positive injection is stopped, K^+ ions will continue to leave the cell, making the interior ever more negative and tend to take the membrane potential back to E_K. In other words, if a cell is permeable to an ion, that is the ion that "responds to perturbations in the equilibrium," and the response is always in the direction of restoring the equilibrium state. This is only natural in a passive system—the cell can only respond with ions that can move through the membrane, the ions to which the cell is selectively permeable.

15. $E_{Na} = 58 \log (150/15)$
    $= 58 \log 10$
    $= 58 (1.00)$
    $= 58$ mV

16. $E_{Na} = 58 \log_{10} (44/50)$, $E_{Na} = 58 \log (15/15)$,
        for squid axon   for mammalian
                                   neuron
    $= 58 \log_{10} 0.88$ $= 58 \log_{10} (1)$
    $= 58 (-0.05)$ $= 58 (0)$
    $= -2.9$ mV $= 0$ mV

The resting potential would probably not be changed at all because the cell is only very slightly permeable to sodium and the resting potential would therefore reflect only a small, if any, change proportional to the degree to which it is permeable to sodium. If any alteration occurred, it would be in the *hyperpolarizing* direction.

17. The membrane potential, V_m, would change to E_{Na}, about +55 mV. The potential would move all the way from –60mV, through 0 mV to +55 mV and remain at this value because (1) it is no longer permeable to K^+ and does not "see" the concentration gradient for this ion and (2) sodium ions would move into the cell, down their concentration gradient, carrying positive charge until enough Na^+ entered the cell to bring the inside to +55 mV. At this point an outward electrical gradient of equal and opposite force would be developed to exactly counter-balance the inward force of the concentration gradient.

18. If you answered "YES" to this question, you are an A-1 biologist, a budding biophysicist, closely related to Sherlock Holmes, and able to read complex sentences with real insight. Congratulations!

19. ATP, Na^+, K^+

20. Ouabain or cooling will reduce the rate of activity of the Na^+, K^+-ATPase ("sodium pump"). The best way to increase its activity is to increase the concentration of

sodium inside the cell or potassium outside—a very nifty design.

21. E_K and E_{Na} are maintained constant.

22. $E_{Cl} = -58 \log_{10}(14/1)$
    $\log_{10}(14/1) = 1.15$
    $E_{Cl} = -58(1.15)$
    $E_{Cl} = -66.5 \text{ mV}$

NOTE: This value is more negative than an average resting potential of around −60mV. This means that if a cell were to become rather selectively permeable to chloride ions, the membrane potential, V_m, would hyperpolarize, right? Right! You are learning!

23. Sodium, potassium.

24. They are spontaneous or endogenous, and they occur rhythmically or regularly.

■ **POST-TEST**

1. The presence of the sodium pump.

2. (a) The Goldman equation accounts for the contribution to the membrane potential of all the different ions to which the membrane is permeable by converting their concentration gradients and relative permeabilities into a composite, "total" electrical potential value.

   (b) Vm =
   $$\frac{RT}{F} \ln \frac{P_K[K^+]_o + P_{Na}[Na^\pm]_o + P_{Cl}[Cl^-]_i}{P_K[K^+]_i + P_{Na}[Na^+]_i + PCl[Cl]_o};$$
   $\frac{RT}{F} \ln$ converts to $58 \log_{10}$ at $25°$ C

   $-65 = 58 \log_{10}$ of
   $$\frac{0.23(20) + P_{Na}(450) + 0.26(40)}{0.23(400) + P_{Na}(50) + 0.26(560)}$$
   Antilog of $-65/58 = 0.076$
   $$0.076 = \frac{4.6 + 450 P_{Na} + 10.4}{92 + 50 P_{Na} + 145.6}$$

$0.076 (92 + 50 P_{Na} + 145.6) =$
$$4.6 + 450 P_{Na} + 10.4$$

$7 + 3.8 P_{Na} + 11.1 =$
$$4.6 + 450 P_{Na} + 10.4$$

$3.1 = 446.2 P_{Na}$

$P_{Na} = 0.007$

$P_{Na}/P_K = 0.007/0.23 = 0.03$

   (c) Yes (in pacemaker cells and during action potentials [see Chapter 3]).

3. The resting potential would initially become more negative (hyperpolarize) if negative current were injected into the cell. Potassium ions would counteract this increased negativity by moving into the cell. Potassium ions would be the most likely ions to do so because they are the ones to which the membrane is most permeable.

4. The membrane potential will approach the *equilibrium potential* for the ion to which it is *permeable*.

5. 10.0 : 0.4 : 4.5 (Or 1 : .04 : .45. Note that a ratio of 0.03 for P_{Na}/P_K was calculated in question 2 above, which is close enough to the 0.04 value here.)

6. V_m is the "generic" term for membrane potential and can be used for any general reference to transmembrane voltage. "Resting membrane potential (RMP)" is only used with specific reference to that condition. E_{ion} refers to the equilibrium potential for a particular ion. Only in the case where a cell were exclusively permeable to one ion and stable at a steady-state value of membrane potential would $V_m = RMP = E_{ion}$.

CHAPTER 3

The Action Potential

Concepts

1. The action potential, or "nerve impulse," is a brief stereotyped change in membrane potential that occurs in excitable cells. An action potential in a typical mammalian neuron goes from the resting potential to a positive value beyond zero potential and back to rest in only 1 to 2 milliseconds (msec).

2. Sodium ions move inward during the earliest phase of an action potential as the cell depolarizes toward the sodium equilibrium potential. Potassium ions then move out of the cell, allowing the inside to return to its negative resting potential near the potassium equilibrium potential.

3. Ohm's law can be used to relate membrane permeability, or conductance, membrane potential and ionic current.

4. The membrane changes its conductances to sodium and potassium ions during an action potential. These conductance (permeability) changes are controlled by the membrane potential.

5. The sodium and potassium ionic current channels involved in the action potential are unique: their conductances are controlled by voltage, and they can be differentiated by their ion selectivity, kinetics, and their behavior in the presence of certain drugs and toxins.

6. The sodium channel and certain other voltage-gated channels for Ca^{++} and K^+ have an activated and an inactivated state.

7. The activity of individual ion channels can be studied by the patch-clamp technique.

The action potential, or nerve impulse, is a brief, stereotyped electrical signal generated by nerve and muscle cells and represents a transient change from the resting state during which the internal potential of the neuron moves from near E_K to a quite positive value and then back to the resting state again. Neurophysiologists hypothesized that the action potential is caused by the membrane becoming suddenly permeable to sodium ions, allowing sodium to run in until the *membrane potential approaches the sodium equilibrium potential* (E_{Na}). E_{Na} has been calculated already to equal about +55 millivolts (mV).

■ SHAPE OF THE ACTION POTENTIAL

A drawing of the parts of an *action potential* and the overall time course of this event are shown in Figure 3-1. During the action potential the transmembrane potential moves rapidly from the resting potential in the depolarizing direction, crosses the zero potential level, and is momentarily reversed in polarity to approximately +30 mV or more (almost to E_{Na}). The part of the spike more positive (or above) zero potential is sometimes called the *overshoot*. The membrane then rapidly repolarizes toward the resting potential. This rapid change in the membrane potential is termed the *spike potential* and occurs in approximately 1 to 2 msec. The decaying (repolarization) phase of the action potential is often followed by a small but relatively long-lasting hyperpolarization beyond the

original resting potential. This is called the *after-hyperpolarization* (AHP) of the action potential; it is variable in amplitude, typically 10 mV or so more negative than the resting potential and may last from a few milliseconds to 100 msec.

■ SODIUM AND POTASSIUM PERMEABILITY CHANGES

What would happen if the resting membrane were made more permeable to sodium? Both the concentration gradient and the membrane potential would tend to move sodium into the cell. There are about ten times more Na^+ ions outside the cell than inside. Even if the transmembrane potential were 0 mV, opening sodium channels would allow the concentration gradient to force Na^+ to the interior and bring the internal potential to a positive value. But in the resting

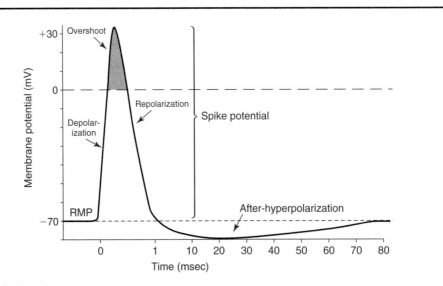

Figure 3-1 ■ Shape and time course of the action potential. For clarity, the first few milliseconds of the time scale have been expanded. Note that the action potential arises from the resting membrane potential (RMP; –70 mV) as a rapidly depolarizing event that carries the internal potential beyond zero to a positive value (the overshoot, shaded area) and then repolarizes again beyond the RMP as an after-hyperpolarization. The size and duration of the after-hyperpolarization can vary among different neurons.

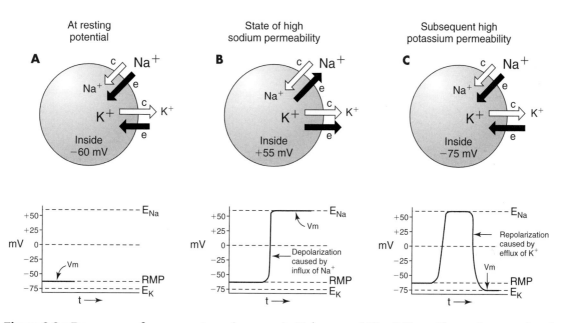

Figure 3-2 ■ **Responses of a neuron to an increase in Na⁺ permeability followed by an increase in K⁺ permeability. A,** At the resting potential (–60 mV), we see the electrical *(e)* and concentration *(c)* gradients acting on Na⁺ and K⁺ ions across the membrane. Recall that at rest, the gradients are nearly equal and opposite for K⁺ ions, but for Na⁺, both the concentration and electrical gradients are directed inward. Below the stylized cell is shown the recorded membrane potential (V_m) of this cell at rest. **B,** When the neuron becomes highly permeable to sodium, these ions would rush into the cell, since initially the concentration and electrical gradients for Na⁺ ions are inward. As sodium enters the cell, the internal potential becomes more and more positive (see recording of V_m below) until the electrical gradient becomes equal and opposite to the inwardly directed concentration gradient. At this point the cell's internal potential would have reached +55 mV, E_{Na}, and will remain there until the permeability to sodium is reduced. Note that because the cell has now achieved an internal potential of +55 mV, the electrical gradient for K⁺ ions is now directed outward, opposite to the situation in the resting state of high internal negativity. **C,** If the neuron were now made highly permeable to K⁺ and impermeable to Na⁺, potassium ions would readily move out of the cell in response to the outwardly directed concentration and electrical gradients. The efflux of K⁺ ions would make the interior of the neuron increasingly negative, and K⁺ ions would leave until the electrical gradient of inward negativity exactly balanced the persistent outward concentration gradient. At that point V_m would be at E_K.

state, the inside of the neuron is actually quite negatively polarized, so the Na⁺ ions will be very strongly attracted to the interior of the cell (Figure 3-2, *A*). Thus an increase in sodium permeability would allow sodium to run passively down its inwardly directed concentration and

electrical gradients and no added energy or work is required. As sodium entered the cell, the internal potential would become more and more positive until the internal positive electrical force was so large that no further net sodium movement into the cell down the concentration gradient could occur. At this point, the outwardly directed electrical force would exactly balance the inwardly directed concentration force and the membrane potential would be at E_{Na} (Figure 3-2, *B*). The membrane potential would be stable at that value unless something else happened. If the membrane were now to stop being permeable to sodium and were to become permeable to potassium instead, what would happen? The concentration gradient, as always, would tend to push potassium ions out of the cell. The electrical gradient would be in the same direction (outward) because the inside of the cell is now positive (Figure 3-2, *B*). Both forces would then cause an efflux of potassium. As potassium left the cell, the inside would become more negative, and this process would go on until the electrical gradient once more exactly balanced the concentration gradient and the membrane potential was at E_K (Figure 3-2, *C*). In this case, we would have returned to near the original resting potential.

At this point, a difficulty frequently arises. During the rising phase (depolarization) of the action potential, the nerve has gained some sodium. During the falling phase (repolarization) it has lost some potassium. Does this mean that the K^+ and Na^+ concentration ratios have changed and, as a result, E_{Na} and E_K have changed? If this were the case, the resting potential and action potential could not maintain their original magnitudes. The answer is that the number of ions necessary to change the membrane potential is extremely small and only negligible changes in internal sodium and potassium concentrations are produced by even a large number of action potentials. This has been demonstrated by measuring fluxes of radiolabeled ions during action potentials where it has been shown that only a few picomoles of sodium cross the membrane during an action potential. We can also gain an idea of the magnitude of sodium ionic current that might move through the membrane during an action potential by a simple calculation based

on electrical considerations. As seen in Chapter 4, nerve cell membranes can be thought of as a form of capacitor, since the lipoidal plasma membrane acts electrically to store coulombs of charge (Q) on its two faces. On average, excitable membranes have been shown to have a capacitance (C) (charge storing capacity) of about 1 μ Farad per square centimeter of membrane surface. The amount of charge (Q) stored on a capacitor can be calculated from the equation

$$Q = CV$$

where V represents the transmembrane potential, i.e., the number of coulombs of charge that can be stored on a capacitor is dependent on the capacitance (C) of the membrane times the membrane potential across the capacitance. If the stored charge is represented by univalent ions, such as Na^+, the number of moles of ion that would move from one side of the membrane to the other during a change in potential can be calculated as

$$moles_{ion} = CV/F$$

where F is the Faraday constant (~10^5 coulombs/mole). If we assume that the total voltage change that occurs during a spike is ~100 mV (10^{-1} volts; the membrane potential changes from –60 mV to +40 mV), then for one cm^2 of membrane

$$moles_{ion} = \frac{10^{-6}\ Farads \times 10^{-1}\ volts}{10^5\ coulombs/mole}$$

$$= 1 \times 10^{-12}\ moles$$

A few more picomoles than this actually move across the membrane during a spike because the charge transfer involves needing extra Na^+ coming in to compensate for the efflux of K^+ that starts to occur near the peak of the action potential. We discuss the ion movements that occur during the action potential in more detail later in this chapter. The important point to remember is that only tiny amounts of ions move across the membrane during an action potential and thus there is no significant change in the intracellular or extracellular ion concentrations. Because the concentrations do not change, there are no significant changes in E_K or E_{Na} during the normal life of a cell. The Na, K-ATPase pump has more than ample capacity to take care of these small shifts in concentration that occur during action potentials and, as pointed out in Chapter 2, can compensate for the even smaller steady-state "leaks" of Na^+ and K^+ ions that occur in the steady-state resting condition of the neuron. *E_K and E_{Na} are constants that are not affected by the normal activity of excitable cells.*

■ **QUESTIONS**   *(Answers at the end of the chapter)*

1. An action potential may be divided into a rapidly occurring _____ and a more slowly occurring _____ .
   The rapidly occurring change of the membrane potential begins with a _____ phase, including an _____ beyond zero potential when the cell becomes positive inside, and this is followed by a phase called _____ during which the potential returns toward the resting level.

2. Which ion is responsible for the current associated with the depolarizing phase of an action potential?

3. Which ion is involved in repolarization?

4. If the resting potential of a cell were –70 mV and the peak of the spike potential were +30 mV, what would the total (absolute) voltage change be for an action potential?

5. If it takes only 0.5 milliseconds for the voltage to change from –70 to +30 mV, what is the rate of change in volts/sec for the depolarizing phase of an action potential?

6. During an action potential, some _____ ions enter the cell and some _____ ions leave the cell. Give two reasons why the nervous system does not "run down."

7. True or false: E_{Na} and E_K remain constant during the normal existence of excitable cells.

8. What is the equilibrium potential for potassium at the peak of the action potential?

■ **CONTROL OF IONIC CONDUCTANCE BY MEMBRANE VOLTAGE**

Up to this point, we have evidence that the permeability to potassium is associated with the resting potential, while a change in sodium permeability might give rise to the action potential. *The key to controlling the membrane potential is the permeability of the membrane, i.e., the membrane potential will be moved toward the equilibrium potential for the ion to which it is most permeable.* The variables that we have been considering are the ionic current and the membrane potential, and it is not immediately obvious how one relates permeability to these. There is a very convenient measure that is proportional to the membrane permeability for an ion, i.e., *conductance*. The conductance, symbolized by the letter g, is the reciprocal of the electrical resistance of a circuit. (Resistance can be thought of as how difficult it is to push current though a circuit; conductance is more or less the opposite—an index of how easily current can move though a circuit.) In a simple circuit with a battery and a resistor the current flow equals the voltage divided by the resistance:

$$I = V/R$$

This simple relationship between current, voltage, and resistance is known as Ohm's law. The conductance, g, is simply the reciprocal of resistance, g = 1/R, and Ohm's law can be rephrased by saying that I = gV. Thus the amount of ionic current (I) that can flow across a membrane will be determined by the conductance (g), or permeability, of the membrane to that ion and by the amount of electrical force (V) there is acting on that ion. The magnitude of the electrical force (V) in our system is actually equivalent to the difference between the membrane potential and the equilibrium potential for the ion. In other words, at its equilibrium potential, there is no net electrical gradient acting on an ion, but if the membrane potential is displaced from the ion's equilibrium potential, then a force is created on the charged ion that is larger the farther the membrane potential is from the equilibrium potential. The ion will move in response to the electrical gradient, or force, in proportion to the degree that the cell is permeable to the ion (g). Thus the conductance of the membrane can be related to electrical driving force and current. The electrical driving force is the difference between the equilibrium potential for an ion (E_{ion}) and the membrane

potential (V_m). Thus a general formula can be written:

$$I_{ion} = g_{ion} (V_m - E_{ion})$$

A large current (I_{ion}) results from a large conductance (g_{ion}) or a large electrical driving force ($V_m - E_{ion}$). This equation is most useful for understanding how voltage, conductance, and ionic currents are interrelated at different times during the normal activity of excitable cells.

What actually controls the permeability or conductance during an action potential? The best way an action potential can be initiated is to reduce the membrane potential. In fact, the factor that controls the conductance is the membrane potential itself. We will assume that decreasing V_m (depolarizing) is going to increase g_{Na}. What will happen? V_m will decrease, and g_{Na} will increase, which will increase the inward movement of Na$^+$ ions (I_{Na} inward). The inward movement of positive ions will further reduce the membrane potential, which in turn produces a further increase in g_{Na}, and so forth. This is a

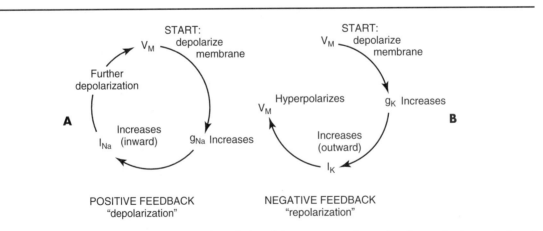

Figure 3-3 ■ **Feedback loops illustrating the relationships among voltage (** V_m **), conductance (** g **) and current (** I **) for Na$^+$ and K$^+$ ions, assuming that the conductance (permeability) for each ion is increased when a neuron is depolarized.**

positive feedback system and is illustrated in Figure 3-3, *A*.

Now, let us see what happens with potassium ions. Assuming that lowering (depolarizing) the membrane potential will also increase g_K, then decreasing V_m leads to an increase in g_K, which leads to an outward movement of K^+ ions (positive I_K outwards has increased because the internal negativity has decreased) and then leads to an increase in V_m. Thus, as the potassium ions move out, there is left an increasing negativity in the cell. In other words, decreasing the membrane potential will tend eventually to bring the membrane potential back to E_K and this, then, will be a process of negative feedback (Figure 3-3, *B*).

The rising phase (depolarization) and the falling phase (repolarization) of the action potential can be quantitatively accounted for by assuming that the conductance to sodium is increased and then decreased, while the conductance to potassium increases at a slower rate.

■ QUESTIONS *(Answers at end of chapter)*

9. What is conductance?

10. (a) Using words, explain what the general formula below means:

$$I_{ion} = g_{ion} (V_m - E_{ion})$$

  (b) On what general electrical law or principle is it based?

  (c) In a resting neuron, the value ($V_m - E_{ion}$) would be the largest for which of the three major ions (Na^+, K^+, Cl^-) that have been discussed?

11. On what membrane electrical characteristic are the conductances of sodium and potassium likely to be dependent during an action potential? Explain the positive feedback loop relating membrane potential, sodium current, and sodium conductance.

12. When positive potassium current leaves a neuron, what happens to the membrane potential?

■ RELATION BETWEEN SODIUM AND POTASSIUM CONDUCTANCE CHANGES AND THE ACTION POTENTIAL–VOLTAGE CLAMP

Can changes in g_{Na} and g_K actually account for the action potential? Are the changes of the proper magnitude and are they timed correctly? What makes these conductances change during the impulse? Two British neurophysiologists, Allen Hodgkin, and Andrew Huxley, set out to determine how g_{Na} and g_K varied with membrane potential and time. They not only managed to solve this problem, but they were also able to reconstruct the action potential in a mathematical model solely by knowledge of these variables. They based their work on a technique called *voltage-clamp,* which was pioneered in the United States by Kenneth Cole. They also chose to do their experiments at the Plymouth marine laboratories where a long history of use of favorable marine specimens for neurophysiological research had revealed the special advantages of the giant axon of the squid.

With the voltage clamp procedure it is possible to hold, or "clamp," the membrane potential electronically at whatever value is desired for many milliseconds with a feedback arrangement and to measure the flow of ionic currents which move across the membrane with that applied voltage change (Figure 3-4). A naturally occurring action potential is so brief that it is impossible to measure changes in conductance or ion flow in any detailed or systematic fashion because Vm is changing so rapidly. With this method, however, it was possible to set and control V_m for a relatively prolonged period (it was also possible to cool the preparation to slow down the processes). The transmembrane current (I_{ion}) was measured directly, and, with the squid axon

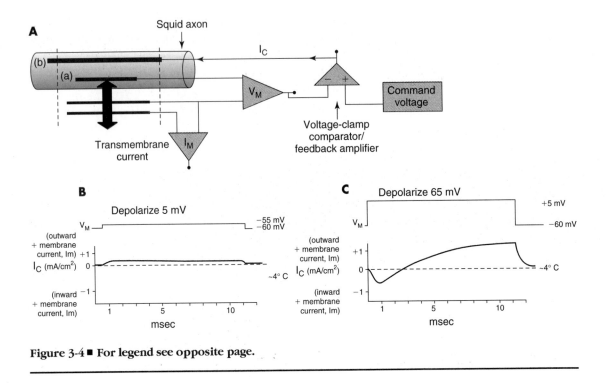

Figure 3-4 ■ For legend see opposite page.

preparation, the concentrations of sodium and potassium, inside and outside, could be controlled and thus E_{Na} and E_K were known and could be altered. With these variables known, the conductance could then be computed [$g_{ion} = I_{ion}/(V_m - E_{ion})$] for any V_m and for any time as well. It was thus possible to determine for any change in membrane potential which ion currents flow and how the conductances to these ions change with voltage and time. The basic results of the classic work of Hodgkin and Huxley are illustrated in Figure 3-5 and described below.

When the membrane potential was depolarized (Figure 3-5, *A*) beyond a certain critical level (threshold), there was a sudden and large inward flow of positive current carried by Na+ ions (Figure 3-5, *B*). The larger the depolarizing step, the greater the current flow on an instantaneous basis. That sodium ions were carrying

this current was proved by changing [Na+]$_o$ and observing that the amount of current flow varied proportionately. There is thus an initial large increase in the conductance (permeability) of the membrane to sodium (Figure 3-5, *C*). This increase in g_{Na} is called *activation*, and the rate of change in g_{Na} is also positively correlated with larger depolarizations—the magnitude and rate of increase of g_{Na} strictly depend on the size of the depolarizing step. When the membrane was clamped in the depolarized state, it was seen (somewhat unexpectedly) that the increased sodium conductance does not persist indefinitely. Another, independent mechanism, which is both voltage- and time-dependent, automatically turns off the sodium conductance, and this process is called *inactivation* (Figure 3-5, *C*).

In addition to the rapid increase and then decay in I_{Na}, it was also found that potassium

Figure 3-4 ■ Schema for voltage-clamp recording from squid axon. A, A several millimeter-long length of a giant axon was placed in a recording chamber (the total amount of surface area of membrane was known). Two wire-electrodes were placed longitudinally into the interior of the axon. One of the wires *(a)* was used for recording membrane potential: amplifier labeled V_m that records difference between interior and exterior of axon. Transmembrane currents (indicated by red arrow crossing the membrane) were recorded *(I_m)* via two extracellular wires that sampled the current flow between them (through the resistance of the surrounding seawater). The length of axon under study was carefully partitioned and electrically isolated *(dotted lines)* so that any current leaving or entering the axon could be accurately sampled. The output of amplifier V_m was fed into a differential feed-back amplifier as a negative input, while command signals, or voltages, were fed into the positive input of the amplifier. The amplifier would then inject an appropriate amount of current *(I_c)* into the axon, via the other intracellular electrode *(b),* to clamp, or hold, V_m at whatever voltage difference between command and V_m that was designated. For example, if the resting potential was at –60 mV and a command signal was given to move V_m to –55 mV (a 5 mV depolarization), then the voltage clamp amplifier would inject enough positive current into the cell to take the potential to –55 mV. The amount of current necessary was measured and plotted as seen in B. A small outward positive current was seen to flow during the period of the clamp. This current would represent the amount of positive current that would have to be placed into the cell to hold the potential at –55 mV in compensation for the passive outward movement of K^+ ions that would occur when the electrical gradient holding them in the cell were reduced by 5 mV (see Figure 2-3, *B*). The power and advantage of the voltage-clamp method is best appreciated, however, when larger command steps are given. C, For example, if the cell is commanded to be depolarized by a large amount, say 65 mV (i.e., move the voltage from rest at –60 mV to +5 mV), this should be more than enough depolarization to open any voltage-gated channels in the membrane. The kinds of current seen now are very different from those resulting from a small depolarization. Note that within a fraction of a millisecond after the voltage is clamped to the depolarized level, there is a large negative current that the amplifier injects into the cell. This is followed after a millisecond by a large and sustained positive current. The currents that are injected into the cell by the voltage-clamp apparatus are compensating for the flow of ions across the neural membrane. The large depolarization opened Na^+ channels and Na^+ ions rushed into the cell. To compensate for this increase in internal positivity (read instantaneously at the V_m amplifier), the voltage-clamp amplifier injected an equal amount of negative charge to hold the potential at the command voltage. Conversely, after the apparent sodium current has peaked, the cell becomes permeable to K^+ ions, which would leave the cell. This outward movement of positive ionic current is compensated by the voltage-clamp apparatus by injecting positive current into the cell at the same rate at which K^+ was leaving. Thus the voltage clamp technique provides a means of accurately monitoring the movement of ionic current into or out of the cell. It should be noted that the sign (+/–) of the current labeled in B and C represents the sign of the current I_c that is injected into the cell by the voltage-clamp comparator/amplifier. Logically and by convention, negative current injected into the cell represents that necessary to compensate for an *inward positive current*, such as influx of Na^+ ions, and such inward-directed positive ionic currents are plotted as going *downward*. Conversely, positive current injected as Ic represents that necessary to compensate for a loss of *positive charge* from the inside of the cell, such as by efflux of K+ ions, and such outward-directed positive ionic currents are plotted as going *upward*.

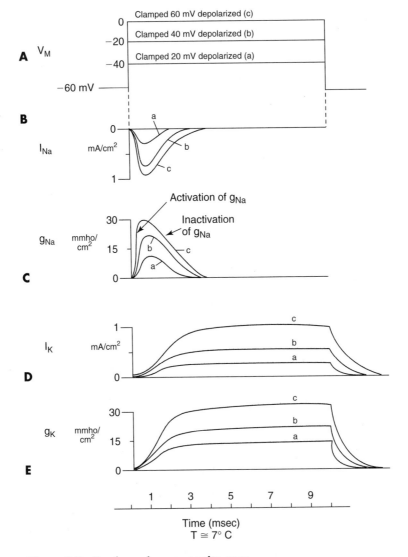

Figure 3-5 ■ For legend see opposite page.

Figure 3-5 ■ Theoretical records from a voltage-clamp experiment in squid axon at 7° C in normal seawater. A illustrates the change in V_m for three different 10-msec voltage-clamp steps, the first *(a)* a 20 mV depolarization, the second *(b)*, 40 mV, and the third *(c)*, 60 mV, each stepped from the resting potential held at –60 mV. The transmembrane currents that flow during each voltage step have been arbitrarily separated into an inward sodium current, I_{Na} (B) and an outward potassium current, I_K (D). (The currents were actually recorded as I_c, the current from the voltage-clamp necessary to move into or out of the cell to maintain the commanded voltage. That such currents reflect the movements of Na^+ or K^+ ions requires showing that the currents are properly influenced by changes in their concentrations or by using compounds or toxins that selectively block specific channels.) Note that the amount of inward Na^+ current increases with depolarization, but that the influx of sodium reaches a peak within a short time and then the current stops. The outward potassium current, on the other hand, while having a magnitude and rate of increase that are also voltage-dependent, continues to flow as long as the depolarizing step is on. When V_m is returned to the resting level, I_K decreases exponentially. The change in conductance for sodium and potassium, calculated from the equation $g_{ion} = I_{ion}/(V_m - E_{ion})$, is plotted in C and E, respectively. As expected, the amount of conductance and its rate of increase are also voltage-dependent: the greater the depolarizing step, the faster g_{Na} and g_K increase. Although not illustrated here, the process of turning off g_{Na} (inactivation) also has voltage- and time-dependence and plays an important role in controlling numerous kinds of voltage-gated channels.

---

current increased with depolarization (Figure 3-5, *D*). There was an outward flow of K^+ ions (positive current) that began shortly after the depolarization was initiated and then persisted throughout the duration of the depolarizing step. The increase in I_K was associated with an increase in g_K (Figure 3-5, *E*) that started with a short delay after the onset of the increase in g_{Na} and was seen to rise more slowly than g_{Na}. The conductance to potassium remains elevated as long as the membrane is held in the depolarized state (Figure 3-5, *E*). Apparently there is not a significant inactivation process for potassium in this preparation. As with g_{Na}, the kinetics of g_K are also voltage-dependent; the rate of increase in g_K increases with larger depolarizations. When the membrane potential is repolarized to the resting level, g_K slowly reverts to its resting value and there is a steady decline in outward K^+ current.

■ **QUESTIONS** *(Answers at end of chapter)*

13. What is the functional advantage of the voltage clamp technique?

14. Besides voltage and time, what other variable can be measured directly with the voltage clamp?

15. How does one obtain a measure of conductance using the voltage clamp?

16. When measuring transmembrane current flow under the conditions we have described, it is not always possible to differentiate between inward flow of positive ions or outward flow of negative ions. The current represented in *B* of Figure 3-5 could be sodium moving inward or it could represent an outward movement of, say, chloride ions. The two currents would "look" the same electrically. How, experimentally and deductively, could you show that the current was carried by sodium and not by chloride?

17. What are sodium activation and inactivation?

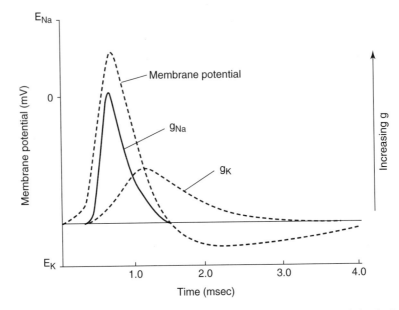

Figure 3-6 ■ **The relationship between the change in membrane potential (V_m) during an action potential and the changes in conductance to sodium (g_{Na}) and potassium (g_K) ions. Note that a large increase in g_{Na} accompanies the depolarization phase of the action potential but that near the peak of the action potential g_{Na} turns off (inactivation); g_K begins to turn on slightly later than does g_{Na}, rises more slowly and declines, without inactivation, to its original resting value as the membrane is repolarized.**

18. If a normal excitable membrane were "clamped" at –10 mV, would gK be greater, less, or the same as when the membrane potential is at rest (–70 mV)?

These results may be organized to explain the full cycle of the action potential (Figure 3-6). With an adequate amount of depolarization, the permeability of the membrane to sodium is increased so that sodium ions rush down their electrochemical gradient, depolarizing the membrane even more. The membrane potential then approaches the sodium equilibrium potential, exactly as outlined earlier. Theoretically, this process would continue until V_m reached E_{Na}. However, there are two membrane mechanisms that prevent this occurrence—one is the inac-

tivation of g_{Na} and the other is the increase in g_K. At the peak of g_{Na}, the membrane is depolarized beyond zero toward E_{Na}. As the membrane now becomes impermeable to sodium (inactivation), it also becomes increasingly permeable to potassium ions; K^+ ions will rush out of the cell (positive current outward), leaving the cell increasingly more negative inside and thus repolarizing it toward E_K. Therefore, it is clear that the rising phase of the spike potential is due to the rapid entry of sodium ions, and the repolarization is due to the outward movement of potassium ions. The after-hyperpolarization is due to a prolonged increase in the potassium conductance, which serves to hold V_m virtually at E_K. The repolarization also turns off the sodium-inactivation mechanism; and after a short period

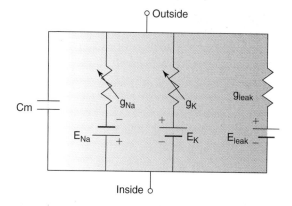

Figure 3-7 ■ **An electrical model of an excitable membrane.** The electrical equivalent of a uniform patch of membrane is shown with four parallel pathways for current to move. Capacitative current can flow onto or away from the membrane capacitance (C_m), and ionic current can cross the membrane through voltage-gated sodium channels or voltage-gated potassium channels. The variable resistances, g_{Na} and g_K, are proportional to the respective permeabilities for these ions, and the conductance increases as the membrane is depolarized. The sodium and potassium batteries are oriented to represent the transmembrane potential sign imposed by the respective equilibrium potentials. A fourth ionic current pathway represents the lumped sum of several non-gated (passive) currents (mainly K$^+$ and Cl$^-$) that move through the membrane via constant, resting conductances (g_{leak}) with a battery that represents the steady-state resting potential.

of time the increase in g_K dies away and the membrane potential returns to its original resting level. The cell is now ready to fire another action potential.

Hodgkin and Huxley formalized an electrical model of the membrane (Figure 3-7) that accounts for the total current that would be involved in an action potential. The model included ionic currents that would flow through voltage gated pores for sodium and potassium, small back-

ground "resting" currents (designated "leak" currents), including those through resting potassium and chloride conductances, and the current that would move at the membrane as capacitative current at the onset of a voltage change. The total current (I_T) that would flow at the membrane during a voltage step would include the capacitative current (I_c) during the voltage change ($C_m(dV_m/dt)$) plus the ionic current that moved through the membrane after the voltage step was constant:

$$I_T = C_m(dV_m/dt) + I_i$$

where C_m is the membrane capacitance, V_m is the size of the voltage step, and I_i is total ionic current comprised of any contributions of sodium (I_{Na}), potassium (I_K), or leak (I_l) currents.

After the voltage change was completed and $dV_m/dt = 0$, then the record of current flow, as in Figure 3-5, *B* and *D*, represented a direct measure of the total ionic flow, and this current could be separated into I_{Na} and I_K components. (The leak currents were negligible and essentially linear and easily subtracted from the major ionic currents.) After the magnitude and time course of I_{Na} and I_K were measured, g_{Na} and g_K could be calculated (see Figure 3-5, *C* and *E*). The truly remarkable contribution of this work, however, came from the production of a series of empirical equations that could be used to describe the complex waveform of the conductance changes over time at any membrane potential. In addition, these equations could be used to calculate and accurately predict the form of an action potential. The underlying hypotheses used to generate the equations were extraordinarily insightful, and features of the equations have proved to be highly applicable to the molecular behavior of channels as discovered with more recent techniques. The two major equations are introduced here, as well as the underlying principles Hodgkin and Huxley used to interpret their form and meaning.

The potassium conductance is given by

$$g_K = \bar{g}_K n^4$$

where $\bar{g}_K$ is a constant equal to the maximum value of g_K. A fourth-order exponential fitted the data rather well, and Hodgkin and Huxley hypothesized that there could be four charged particles that had to change position in the membrane under the influence of the electric field in order for K^+ ions to be able to move through the membrane. The quantity n was the probability that one of these particles was in the correct position. Further equations with rate constants, themselves voltage-dependent, were developed to describe the changes in n with time. In a comparable way, an empirical formula describing the sodium conductance was developed, where $g_{Na} = \bar{g}_{Na} m^3 h$. Again, $\bar{g}_{Na}$ is a constant equivalent to maximum g_{Na}; m is the probability that a hypothetical membrane particle, of which there might be three, is in a correct location in the membrane for permitting Na^+ flow, and $(1-h)$ is the probability that such a particle is inactivated. Additional equations to describe rate constants and voltage-dependencies for m and h had to be developed as well. These equations described quite accurately the behavior of g_K and g_{Na} during an action potential. Whether or not there may be "particles" is an open question; but, in fact, the conceptual model and mathematical description of channel opening by changes in the transmembrane electrical field that displace intramembrane charges has had direct applicability to more recent molecular models of ion channels. Certain transmembrane stretches (the S4 segment, see section on voltage-gated channels) of voltage-dependent ion channel proteins contain charged amino acids, and these parts of the molecule change position within the membrane with depolarization, inducing a conformational change in the channel that permits ion flow. This segment 4 of the channel molecule is termed a *gate,* and it is even possible to record gating currents produced by the movements of the charged amino acids in the membrane.

Since these early experiments at mid-century, rapid advances in technology have permitted the application of voltage-clamp procedures to the study of the properties of virtually any nerve cell. Transistors, microcircuits, and computers, as well as the advent of glass microelectrodes (see Figure 2-1), have made it much simpler to voltage clamp even quite small neurons. Instead of using thin insulated wires for electrodes and thus being restricted to using large-diameter "giant" axons, it became possible to impale smaller cells with microelectrodes and connect them to more rapidly functioning and versatile voltage-clamping devices. Of even greater utility was the development of another means of recording from cells called the patch-clamp technique (Figure 3-8). Invented by Erwin Neher and Bert Sakmann, this technique uses glass micropipettes similar in shape and dimensions to sharp microelectrodes. In this case the tip of the microelectrode is fire-polished to a very smooth finish, and the electrode is brought onto the surface of the cell instead of being inserted into the cell. A small amount of suction is used to attach the tip of the pipette to the cell surface. A very tight seal of high electrical resistance is formed between the electrode tip and the cell membrane. The tiny patch of membrane encircled by the electrode tip can be ruptured to create continuity between the cytoplasm and the electrolyte solution within the electrode barrel. The electrode has accessed the interior of the cell, and the intracellular potential can be recorded by this so-called whole-cell recording technique. Even more remarkably, patch electrodes can be used to record the current flowing through single ion channels within a patch of membrane isolated by the electrode seal. Thus even the behavior of single channels can be monitored and the opening of channels by changes in voltage or by the effects of synaptic

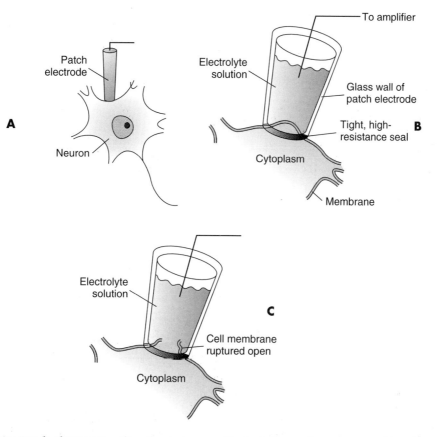

Figure 3-8 ■ Patch-clamp recording from nerve cells. A, A glass micropipette with a smoothed tip can be brought into contact with the surface of a neuron. The electrode is filled with an electrolyte solution that approximates the ionic composition of the cell cytoplasm. **B,** The microelectrode is pressed gently onto the surface of the cell, which if possible has been "cleaned" of nearby glial membrane and other "debris," and slight negative pressure is applied to the back of the electrode. This can cause the tip surface of the electrode to adhere tightly to the cell membrane and the patch of membrane blebs into the interior of the electrode tip. **C,** The patch of membrane within the electrode tip can be ruptured or torn so that the cytoplasm of the neuron is continuous with the electrolyte solution in the electrode barrel. This forms a low-resistance pathway to the interior of the cell surrounded by a high-resistance seal between the edge of the electrode and the cell surface. Intracellular recording from the neuron is now possible, and the membrane potential can be voltage-clamped as well. This manner of recording membrane potentials with patch electrodes is called *whole-cell* patch recording. Patch electrodes can also be used to record the currents that flow through even a single channel that might reside in the patch of membrane at the tip of the electrode (see Figure 3-10).

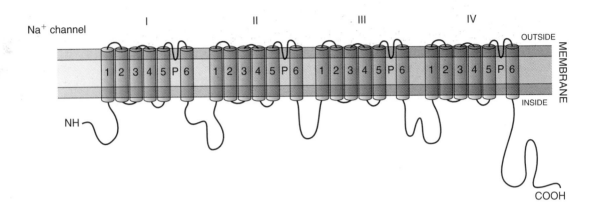

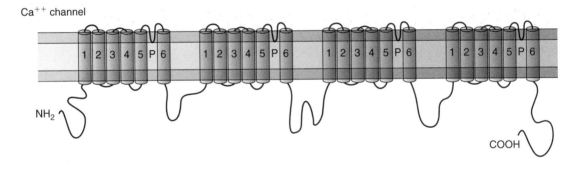

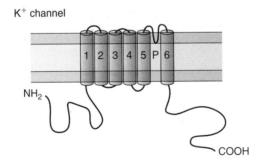

Figure 3-9 ■ **For legend see opposite page.**

Figure 3-9 ■ The structure of voltage-gated ion channels. The voltage-gated sodium channel is believed to be formed by a single, large protein (the alpha subunit) shown here. The protein has four highly homologous domains *(I-IV)*, each containing six transmembrane α-helices numbered *segments 1-6*. A span of amino acids (the *P loop*) between *segments 5 and 6* is believed to contribute to the ion selectivity of the hydrophilic pore of the channel. *Segment 4* is believed to be involved in the voltage-sensing function (gating) of the channel protein and to shift outward slightly in its location in the membrane during a depolarization of the membrane electric field; this induces a conformational change in the other parts of the molecule to open the channel. The natural configuration of the channel involves a conformational clustering of the four domains so as to create a hydrophilic pore whose walls and selectivity filter are formed by subsets of the α-helices and P loops. Certain extracellular stretches of amino acids between segments are known to be binding sites for toxins, such as TTX, and particular intracellular loops are believed to contribute to the inactivation process by moving to block the channel with strong depolarization. Voltage-gated calcium channels are very similar to the sodium channels, differing by only a few amino acids. The voltage-gated potassium channel is formed by a single protein that is equivalent to one of the four repeating domains of sodium and calcium channels. Four of these K^+-channel proteins assemble together to form the functional potassium channel. The strong homology among the domains is part of the evidence for believing that the Ca^{++} and Na^+ channels are descendants of an original K^+-type channel, which was extended by simple gene duplication. An ancient kinship among all K^+-selective channels is suggested by the fact that potassium channels such as those involved in establishing the resting potential and other K^+ channels in prokaryotes (see Figure 2-7) also share homologies with *segments 5 and 6* and the interconnecting P loop in more modern voltage-gated K^+ channels.

---

transmitters can be investigated (see later section and Figure 3-10).

■ **QUESTIONS** *(Answers at end of chapter)*

19. Why doesn't the membrane potential just stay at E_{Na} when an action potential occurs?

20. What conductance changes cause the rising phase of the spike potential, the falling phase, the after-hyperpolarization?

21. Give examples of ways the duration of the squid axon action potential might be altered.

22. Draw a simple graph illustrating the relationship of the conductance changes to sodium and potassium and the voltage change of the action potential over time.

About how long does an action potential last?

23. What is the major functional consequence of the sodium inactivation mechanism?

■ **THE MACROSCOPIC FLOW OF IONS DURING THE ACTION POTENTIAL IS CARRIED OUT BY DISCRETE VOLTAGE-GATED CHANNELS**

In the previous chapter we introduced ion-selective channels, integral membrane proteins composed of transmembrane α-helices with intra- and extracellular loops or spans of amino acid residues between them that could assemble in the membrane and allow K^+ ions to move through them (see Figure 2-7). In addition to those channels that subserve the resting perme-ability to potassium ions, there is a large family of other channels that are also ion selective, but whose molecular structure is influenced by the membrane potential so that depolarization of the membrane actually causes the channels to open. These *voltage-gated channels* belong to a family of genes that are quite similar to one another and are likely descended from an ancient potassium-selective channel gene that gave rise to a line becoming modern voltage-sensitive K^+ channels. First, Ca^{++}-selective and more recently Na^+-selective voltage-gated channel genes arose from the K^+-channel genes. These three protein subfamilies, although having remarkable fidelity of selection for their respective ion species, are homologous and share a similar pattern of at least secondary protein structure (Figure 3-9). There are large numbers of different types of voltage-gated K^+ channels, numerous types of Ca^{++} channels, and a few types of Na^+ channels. The term *types* means that various channel proteins have different functional properties because they have slightly different amino acid sequences. Each channel may open or close with a different voltage sensitivity or at different rates (i.e., different channels have different kinetics); some channels have an inactivation state, others do not; some permit ion flow more readily in one direction across the membrane than another (rectification); some channel types may be expressed at different times in development or in response to certain types of injury or pathological change; some channel proteins have associated with them other membrane proteins that can modulate their function.

Different neurons and muscle cells express different members of the various subfamilies, and they insert the various channels at strategic locations on their membrane surface as we discuss in greater details in later chapters. In general, any particular nerve cell expresses a rich variety of kinds of channels, and their properties can have significant impact on nerve cell behavior. For example, the action potential seen in the squid giant axon is produced by the fairly ubiquitous voltage-gated Na^+ channel seen in most neurons, whereas the repolarization of the action potential is produced by efflux of K^+ ions through a voltage-gated potassium channel called the *delayed rectifier.* (The term *delayed* is used because the channel opens with a slight delay after the sodium channels start to open, and *rectifier* is used because the channel readily permits K^+ ion efflux through it but does not easily pass K^+ in the inward direction). The voltage-dependence and kinetics of these two channel types confer a certain consistent "signature" or waveform to the squid axon action potential. In many other neurons a different type of voltage-dependent K^+ channel may participate in action potential repolarization. The properties of these channels could confer a different shape on the action potential: it might repolarize faster or lack a significant after-hyperpolarization. This could mean that such neurons could fire action potentials at a higher frequency because the increase in potassium conductance associated with repolarization persists for a shorter time.

Finally, different types of channels can be blocked quite selectively by a variety of kinds of natural toxins and other compounds. For example, the voltage-sensitive sodium channels responsible for the depolarizing phase of the action potential are selectively blocked by tetrodotoxin (TTX—a poison from puffer fish) and by saxitoxin and related compounds from certain dinoflagellates. Sodium channels can also be blocked by lidocaine, procaine (Novocain), cocaine, and other esters of benzoic acid that are used as local anesthetics, but the affinity and selectivity of these compounds for the sodium channel are less than those of the toxins. Certain voltage-sensitive potassium channels, including the so-called delayed rectifier that is responsible for action potential repolarization in squid axon, can be selectively blocked by the cation tetraethylammonium (TEA). Other K^+ channels are blocked fairly selectively by different chemicals and toxins. There are at least four distinct types of Ca^{++}-selective voltage-gated channels (the so-called T, N, L, and P/Q types) that differ in their kinetics, whether and how they are inactivated, and in their physiological roles in neurons. These channels can be selectively blocked by several types of toxins or by other divalent ions, such as Mg^{++}, Cd^{++} or Co^{++}, that are too large to go through the Ca^{++} channel and "plug" it.

Such toxins and blocking agents have been invaluable tools to help sort out the contributions of various voltage-gated channels and their respective ionic currents during action potentials, especially when use of the toxins is combined with voltage-clamp studies so that particular currents can be isolated (by blocking other currents) and characterized. Another important means by which voltage-gated channels have been studied is by patch-clamp recording of single channels (Figure 3-10). It is possible to record the ionic current flow through a single channel (or a very few channels) that has been electrically isolated in a patch of membrane under a patch electrode. The patch of membrane containing the isolated channel can be clamped at various potentials and the behavior of the channel can be recorded. The major features of voltage-gated channels that have been studied in this way include the following. The opening of channels is indeed voltage-dependent; the probability of a channel opening is greater the greater the amount of depolarization applied across the membrane. Channel opening and closing is an "all-or-nothing" event—when depolarization is applied the channels open to pass a discrete amount of current and then the channel closes. Each channel type has a single-channel conductance that follows ohmic relations, i.e., the amount of current passed for a particular amount of voltage change is constant: $g_{channel} = I_{channel}/(V_m-E_{ion})$. TTX-sensitive sodium channels have a single-channel conductance of about 10 to 20 picosiemens. ("Siemens" is the unit for

conductance and is simply the inverse of resistance, 1/ohms, sometimes written as "mho.") Most voltage-dependent K^+ channels have single-channel conductances in this same range, although certain K^+ channels have higher conductances. Voltage-dependent Ca^{++} channels are more difficult to study but probably in general have somewhat lower single-channel conductances. The behavior of individual channels can be accurately extrapolated, based on their voltage sensitivity, conductance, open-times, and density in the membrane, to account for the macroscopic currents that are seen in a whole cell with voltage clamping and the behavior of whole-cell currents as described mathematically by Hodgkin and Huxley.

■ **QUESTIONS** *(Answers at the end of the chapter)*

24. List three major features of the channels involved with action potential currents.

25. Are voltage-dependent channels selective about *direction* of ion flow through them?

26. What are some major differences between the voltage-dependent sodium and potassium channels?

27. Because voltage-gated channels do not directly employ metabolic energy to allow ions to pass through the membrane, why do you think excitable tissues have such high metabolic rates?

■ **POST-TEST**

1. Would the peak of the after-hyperpolarization of the action potential be more or less negative than normal when external potassium concentration is decreased?

2. What controls membrane potential? What controls membrane permeability?

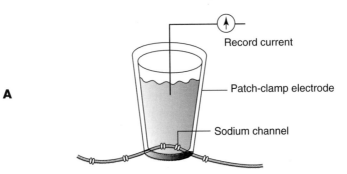

A

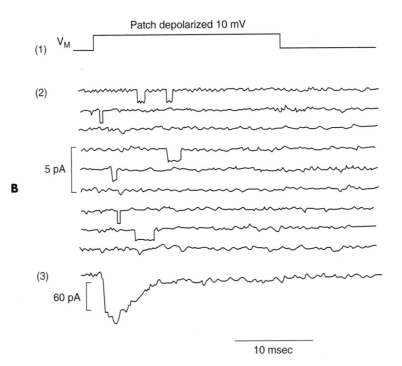

Patch depolarized 10 mV

(1) V_M

(2)

5 pA

B

(3)

60 pA

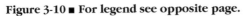

10 msec

Figure 3-10 ■ For legend see opposite page.

Figure 3-10 ■ **The patch-clamp technique can be used to record the current flowing through single voltage-dependent sodium channels. A, A patch electrode isolates a few sodium channels whose individual openings can be detected as small pulses of current that flow when the patch of membrane is depolarized. B, Sample records from an experiment in which the membrane patch was depolarized by 10 mV** *(1)* **on 300 separate trials and the current flow through the channels within the patch was recorded—sample traces from individual trials are shown in** *(2)*. **Each downward "square-wave" represents a discrete pulse of inward sodium current that occurs when the channel is open. Note that the channels tend to open near the beginning of the depolarizing step and that they remain open only a brief time (average open time here was 0.7 msec) because they inactivate shortly after opening. The average amount of peak sodium current that flowed in each channel opening was 1.6 pA. Single-channel conductance was calculated to be 18 pS. The bottom trace** *(3)* **represents the sum of the individual current events captured in the set of 300 trials represented in** *(2)*. **The time course of the total current (as well as the average time course of individual events) indicates that the statistical behavior of a population of channels mimics the time course of total membrane sodium current during depolarization, with most channels opening within the first 1 or 2 msec and decaying with an overall time constant consistent with that for inactivation of the sodium current in an intact cell.** (Adapted from Nicholls JG, Martin AR, Wallace BG, et al: *From neuron to brain*, ed 4, Sunderland, Mass, 2001, Sinauer Associates; Sigworth FJ, Neher E: Single Na$^+$ channel currents observed in cultured rat muscle cells, *Nature* 287:447-449, 1980.)

---

3. Is it true that if the membrane potential of a normal neuron were clamped at +100 mV, sodium ions would leave the cell? Explain why.

4. If the membrane potential were hyperpolarized a few mV negative to the resting potential, in what way would you expect voltage-gated channel conductances to change?

5. Why are action potentials referred to as "all-or-nothing" electrical events?

■ **REFERENCES AND ADDITIONAL READINGS**

Aidley DJ: *The physiology of excitable cells*, ed 4, Cambridge, 1998, Cambridge University Press.

Aidley DJ, Stanfield PR: *Ions channels: molecules in action*, Cambridge, 1996, Cambridge University Press.

Anderson OS, Koeppe RE: Molecular determinants of channel function, *Physiol Rev* 72 (suppl):S89-S158, 1992.

Armstrong CM: Voltage-dependent ionic channels and their gating, *Physiol Rev* 72 (suppl):S5-S13, 1992.

Armstrong CM, Hille B: Voltage-gated ion channels and electrical excitability, *Neuron* 20:371-380, 1998.

Bean BP: Classes of calcium channels in vertebrate cells, *Annu Rev Physiol* 51:367-384, 1989.

Birnbaumer L, Campbell KP, Catterall WA, et al: The naming of voltage-gated calcium channels, *Neuron* 13:505-506, 1994.

Catterall WA: Cellular and molecular biology of voltage-gated sodium channels, *Physiol Rev* 72(suppl):S15-S48, 1992.

Catterall WA: Structure and function of voltage-gated ion channels, *Annu Rev Biochem* 64:493-531, 1995.

Chandy KG, Gutman GA: Voltage-gated potassium channel genes. In North A (ed): *Ligand- and voltage-gated channels*, Boca Raton, Fla, 1995, CRC Press, pp 1-72.

Cole KS, Curtis HJ: Electrical impedance of the squid giant axon during activity, *J Gen Physiol* 22:649-670, 1939.

Connor JA, Stevens CF: Voltage clamp studies of a transient outward membrane current in gastropod neural somata, *J Physiol* (London) 213:21-30, 1971.

Fox AP, Nowycky MC, Tsien RW: Kinetic and pharmacological properties distinguishing three types of calcium currents in chick sensory neurons, *J Physiol* (London) 394:149-172, 1987.

Hamill OP, Marty A, Neher E, et al: Improved patch-clamp techniques for high-resolution current recording from cells and cell-free membrane patches, *Pflugers Arch* 391:85-100, 1981.

Heinemann SH, Terlau H, Stuhmer W, et al: Calcium channel characteristics conferred on the sodium channel by single mutations, *Nature* 356:441-443, 1992.

Hille B: *Ionic channels of excitable membranes*, ed 2, Sunderland, Mass, 1992, Sinauer Associates.

Hodgkin AL, Huxley AF: Currents carried by sodium and potassium ions through the membrane of the giant axon of *Loligo, J Physiol* (London) 116:449-472, 1952.

Hodgkin AL, Huxley AF: The components of membrane conductance in the giant axon of *Loligo, J Physiol* (London) 116:473-496, 1952.

Hodgkin AL, Huxley AF: The dual effect of membrane potential on sodium conductance in the giant axon of *Loligo, J Physiol* (London) 116:497-506, 1952.

Hodgkin AL, Huxley AF: A quantitative description of membrane current and its application to conduction and excitation in nerve, *J Physiol* (London) 117:500-544, 1952.

Hodgkin AL, Huxley AF, Katz B: Measurement of current-voltage relations in the membrane of the giant axon of *Loligo, J Physiol* (London) 116:424-448, 1952.

Hodgkin AL, Katz B: The effect of sodium ions on the electrical activity of the giant axon of the squid, *J Physiol* (London) 108:37-77, 1949.

Huguenard J, McCormick DA: *Electrophysiology of the neuron*, New York, 1994, Oxford University Press.

Jan LY, Jan YN: How might the diversity of potassium channels be generated? *Trends Neurosci* 13:415-419, 1990.

Jan LY, Jan YN: Cloned potassium channels from eucaryotes and prokaryotes, *Annu Rev Neurosci* 20:91-123, 1997.

Keynes RD: The ionic movements during nervous activity, *J Physiol* (London) 114:119-150, 1951.

Kukuljan M, Labarca P, Latorre R: Molecular determinants of ion conduction and inactivation of K+ channels, *Am J Physiol* 268:C535-C556, 1995.

Latorre R, Oberhauser A, Labarca P, et al: Varieties of calcium-activated potassium channels, *Annu Rev Physiol* 51: 385-399, 1989.

Llinas RR: The intrinsic electrophysiological properties of mammalian neurons: insights into central nervous system function, *Science* 242:1654-1664, 1988.

Maubecin VA, Sanchez VN, Siri MDR, et al: Pharmacological characterization of the voltage-dependent Ca2+ channels present in synaptosomes from rat and chicken central nervous system, *J Neurochem* 64:2544-2551, 1995.

McCormick DA: Membrane potential and action potential. In Zigmond MJ et al (eds): *Fundamental neuroscience*, New York, 1999, Academic Press, pp 129-154.

Meech RW, Standen NB: Potassium activation in *Helix aspersa* neurones under voltage clamp: a component mediated by calcium influx, *J Physiol* (London) 249:211-239, 1975.

Miller C: Genetic manipulation of ion channels: a new approach to structure and mechanism, *Neuron* 2:1195-1205, 1989.

Narahashi T, Moore JW, Scott WR: Tetrodotoxin blockage of sodium conductance increase in lobster giant axons, *J Gen Physiol* 47:965-974, 1964.

Neher E, Sakmann B: Single-channel currents recorded from membrane of denervated frog muscle fibers, *Nature* 260: 799-802, 1976.

Nicholls JG, Martin AR, Wallace BG, et al: *From neuron to brain*, ed 4, Sunderland, Mass, 2001, Sinauer Associates.

Noda M, Shimizu S, Tanabe T, et al: Primary structure of *Electrophorus electricus* sodium channel deduced from cDNA sequence, *Nature* 312:121-127, 1984.

Novakovic SD, Eglen RM, Hunter JC: Regulation of Na+ channel distribution in the nervous system, *Trends Neurosci* 24:473-478, 2001.

Nowycky MC, Fox AP, Tsien RW: Three types of neuronal calcium channel with different calcium agonist sensitivity, *Nature* 316:440-443, 1985.

Rudy B, McBain CJ: Kv3 channels: voltage-gated K+ channels designed for high-frequency repetitive firing, *Trends Neurosci* 24:517-526, 2001.

Salkoff L, Baker K, Butler A, et al: An essential "set" of K+ channels conserved in flies, mice and humans, *Trends Neurosci* 15:161-166, 1992.

Sigworth FJ, Neher E: Single Na+ channel currents observed in cultured rat muscle cells, *Nature* 287:447-449, 1980.

Stuhmer W, Conti F, Suzuki H, et al: Structural parts involved in activation and inactivation of the sodium channel, *Nature* 339:597-603, 1989.

Tsien RW, Lipscombe D, Madison DV, et al: Multiple types of neuronal calcium channels and their selective modulation, *Trends Neurosci* 11:431-438, 1988.

■ ANSWERS
Text Questions

1. Spike potential; after-hyperpolarization; depolarizing; over-shoot; repolarization.

2. Sodium

3. Potassium

4. 100 mV

5. 200 volts/sec: 100 mV/0.5 msec = 0.IV/.0005 sec = 1000 V/5secs = 200 V/sec

6. Sodium; potassium. (1) Relatively speaking, only a tiny number of ions of sodium or potassium move across the membrane during an action potential. Recall that the normal intracellular and extracellular

concentrations for these ions is in the mM (i.e., 10^{-3} M) range. Only a few picomoles (10^{-12} M) of ions move across the membrane during a spike. This was proven indirectly by calculating the net amount of charge that would have to move across a membrane having the capacitance of an excitable cell and knowing that one mole of ions has 96,500 coulombs of charge (Faraday's number). The movements of ions was measured directly as well, using radioactive tracers. (2) The sodium pump is able to transport the sodium back out and the potassium back into the cell with ease.

7. True

8. The same as at the resting potential or at any other time, –75 mV (see question 7).

9. Conductance (g) is a measure of membrane permeability for a particular ion. It is an electrical term, the reciprocal of resistance, and thus may be used quantitatively in solutions of Ohm's law.

10. (a) The formula says that the amount of ionic current that will flow through the membrane is dependent on two variables: (1) the permeability or conductance of the membrane and (2) the electrical driving force on the ion created by the difference between the membrane potential and the equilibrium potential for that ion (at which no net ionic current will flow).
    (b) Ohm's law: V = IR.
    (c) Sodium (–70 –[+55]) = –125 mV.

11. Membrane potential. Depolarization of the membrane potential automatically turns on sodium conductance, allowing sodium to move across the membrane to reach electrochemical equilibrium. Sodium ions then move into the cell in response to their concentration and potential gradients; this increase in internal positive sodium ions in turn depolarizes the cell more (makes it more positive inside) and this turns on g_{Na} more, allowing more sodium ion current in, etc.

12. The membrane potential hyperpolarizes or becomes more negative.

13. The voltage-clamp technique, thanks to the electronic circuitry it employs, enables the investigator to hold a variable (voltage) constant while examining that variable's effect on another parameter (current). The normal action potential occurs much too rapidly (remember question 5?), and its waveform is too complex to allow a detailed analysis of its underlying mechanisms. The voltage clamp provides the quantitative control of membrane potential necessary to explore these biophysical events.

14. Transmembrane current. The net flow of current across the squid axon membrane was measured by electrodes outside the axon.

15. The values for conductance were obtained indirectly (and tediously) by Hodgkin and Huxley by calculation using the basic formula: $g = I/(V_m – E)$; they did not have computers. I and V_m were measured directly. E, the equilibrium potential for the appropriate ion, was obtained by direct measurement of intracellular and extracellular concentrations of the ion and using the Nernst equation; g had to be

calculated for many different voltages (depending on where V_m was clamped) and at varying times (e.g., 0.1 msec, 0.5 msec, 1 msec, etc).

16. The reasoning one could use to deduce that the depolarizing phase of the action potential is caused by an inward sodium current and not by an outward chloride current is actually very straightforward: when the membrane is clamped, as in Figure 3-5, with the inside of the cell more positive than the normal resting potential, a very attractive (+) environment would be created for chloride ions, which are negatively charged. Thus, if there were a flow of chloride ions, they would move inward, not outward, with depolarization of the membrane. (Incidentally, it is known that chloride conductance does not change during the action potential.) The experimental proof that sodium moves into the cell during an action potential has been suggested already: change the extracellular sodium ion concentration $[Na^+]_o$ and see if the amount of inward current varies at different voltages. Early investigators had shown that the peak of the spike potential (or the overshoot) was reduced if $[Na^+]_o$ was reduced. Essentially the same experiment can be done with the voltage clamp. When $[Na^+]_o$ is reduced, E_{Na} becomes less positive (check this out with the Nernst equation). If $[Na^+]_o$ is reduced by 50%, E_{Na} for the squid axon will drop from +55 mV to about +37 mV. This means the driving force, or electrical gradient ($V_m - E_{Na}$) will be less than normal at every membrane potential. Thus, the amount of inward sodium current is reduced under this condition for all the values at which you clamp the membrane. Furthermore, in normal seawater, when you clamp the

membrane to potentials (V_m) nearer and nearer E_{Na}, you also reduce the driving force on sodium. If you clamped the membrane at +55 mV so that $V_m = E_{Na}$, then there would be no electrical driving force on sodium and thus no inward current. By using varying amounts of $[Na^+]_o$ and by clamping to several values of V_m with respect to E_{Na}, you could produce a family of current curves whose magnitude and direction would match only the logical behavior of sodium ions based on the Nernst equation and the formula, $I_{Na} = g_{Na} (V_m - E_{Na})$.

17. *Sodium activation* is the term used to define the turning on of sodium conductance by membrane depolarization. It is a process comparable to potassium activation except that it is more sensitive to voltage and turns on very rapidly. Sodium inactivation is a process that is opposite to sodium activation and totally independently controlled. It represents an "active" turning off of sodium conductance. The activation process just gets started when this separate, independent process turns the permeability to sodium back off again. Activation opens the sodium channels quickly by a voltage- and time-dependent mechanism that is begun with only a small delay after the membrane is depolarized; the same depolarization switches on the inactivation mechanism only slightly later and this closes the channel.

18. g_K would be greater.

19. The sodium inactivation mechanism is turned on, and this leads to a decrease in g_{Na}; also g_K is turned on and drives the cell back toward E_K.

20. The rising phase of the spike potential is

caused by an increased g_{Na}; the falling phase by an increase in g_K and a decrease in g_{Na} (sodium inactivation). The after-hyperpolarization is caused by a relatively long and exclusive increase in g_K that outlasts the repolarization period.

21. (a) Change in rate of turn-on of g_{Na}; (b) change in rate of turn-on of sodium inactivation mechanism; or (c) change in rate of turn-on of g_K.

22. The graph should resemble Figure 3-6. The spike potential normally has a duration of around 0.5 to 2 msec. The entire action potential, including the after-hyperpolarization, may be 100 msec long.

23. It allows complete repolarization of the action potential to occur (by turning off g_{Na}).

24. The most important feature of the sodium and potassium channels that operate during the action potential is that their conductance is voltage-dependent. Also, each of the channels is selective for its own ion, mainly because of the size and charge of the channel opening. Finally, these channels are highly selectively blocked by specific agents: tetrodotoxin blocks the sodium channel; tetraethylammonium blocks the potassium channel.

25. No, generally the directionality of flow is determined by the concentration and electrical gradients acting on the ions, although some K^+ channels particularly are known to be rectifying channels that facilitate ion movement better in one direction than the other, either inward or outward.

26. Besides being selective for its own ion and

having different blocking agents, these two channels differ mainly in that in general the potassium channel does not have an inactivation mechanism. It has kinetics of voltage-dependence that make it turn-on more slowly and with a delay compared to the sodium channel.

27. A great deal of energy is required by excitable cells to fuel the sodium pump and other ion pumps, which are continuously busy keeping ion concentrations constant. Also, energy is needed, as in other cells, to maintain pH and proper osmotic balances. Finally, nerve cells are extremely active chemical factories, constantly manufacturing new axoplasm, chemical transmitters, or hormones for release at their axon terminals.

■ POST-TEST

1. The peak of the after-hyperpolarization would be more negative in the presence of decreased external potassium because the equilibrium potential for potassium would be more negative.

2. Permeability; membrane potential.

3. Yes. If V_m were clamped at +100 mV, the membrane potential would be even more positive than E_{Na} (+55 mV). Therefore the inside of the cell would be positive enough to repel the internal sodium ions. This electrical driving force is strong enough to overcome the concentration gradient, and sodium ions would move from the inside to the outside of the cell.

4. They would become less than normal. Voltage-dependence works for depolarization *and* hyperpolarization.

5. Because they are stereotyped, unitary

events of virtually constant size and duration whose underlying causes are automatic regenerative events that depend on the functional properties of channel molecules. Even more fundamentally, one could say this is true because E_{Na} and E_K are held constant. The built-in properties of the membrane are such that the voltage-dependent conductance changes simply switch the cell from a state of high g_K to one of high g_{Na} and back to high g_K. Since the membrane potential moves to the equilibrium potential for the ion to which it is most permeable and since E_{Na} and E_K are constant, the action potential has constant limits of size and shape. Action potentials in different cells can take on different forms, however. In some cells, Ca^{++} channels may contribute to the depolarization of the action potential, and because of the difference in kinetics of such channels compared to the voltage-dependent Na^+ channel, the rise time and height of the spike may be altered. Also, many neurons utilize a variety of types of K^+ channels for repolarization; and thus the rate of repolarization or size of the AHP may be different—action potentials can be longer or shorter in duration and may be repeated more rapidly or fire in bursts.

CHAPTER 4

Excitability, Local Responses, and Passive Electrical Properties of Membranes

Concepts

1. Nerve cell membranes undergo certain relatively small voltage fluctuations, either positive or negative, that are called *local responses*. These are subthreshold, graded potential changes that can summate and alter the excitability of nerve cells. Synaptic potentials and sensory receptor potentials are examples of naturally occurring local responses.

2. Threshold is the membrane potential value (depolarized, or more positive, than the resting potential) at which an action potential is generated. The "excitability" of a neuron—how easily an action potential can be triggered—is inversely related to threshold. Most neurons have a certain part of their membrane, a "trigger zone," that has an especially low threshold or high excitability.

3. During an action potential the cell undergoes three major phases of excitability: (a) absolutely refractory period, (b) relatively refractory period, and (c) subnormal period.

4. Accommodation is a state of greatly reduced excitability (high threshold) induced by prolonged depolarization and a concomitant inactivation of sodium channels.

5. Whereas cytoplasm and extracellular fluid have relative low resistance (r_i, r_o, respectively) to current flow, the membrane has a very high resistance (R_m) and a relatively high capacitance (C_m). The membrane in its passive, resting state behaves like an RC circuit: an electrical circuit with a resistor and capacitor in parallel. This means that the currents associated with local responses are relatively slow, occur on an exponential time scale, and dissipate quickly as they flow away from their point of origin.

6. The time course of local currents can be characterized by a time constant, τ ($= r_m c_m$). The distribution of the passive voltage change over the space of the membrane can be described by a length constant, λ ($= \sqrt{r_m/(r_i + r_o)}$). The time and length constants give the time or distance, respectively, that any local response in a cell will take to decrement to $1/e$ ($\sim 1/3$ or 37%) of its original size.

7. Because of the nature of local responses, neurons constantly integrate all incoming synaptic signals and the membrane potential will fluctuate until threshold is reached at the trigger zone where an action potential is set off.

8. Receptor potentials are a kind of local response produced by the endings of certain sensory neurons.

The previous chapters have considered the ionic basis of the resting potential and the action potential, examining in detail the special relationship of voltage and conductance in these membrane states. This chapter examines an even more fundamental characteristic of a membrane, i.e., a membrane's electrical properties. The membranes of all excitable cells have passive electrical characteristics that are very similar to those of long, insulated electrical cables and are sometimes referred to as *cable* or *electrotonic* properties. These characteristics are different from the active membrane events that cause an action potential, but it is these underlying electrotonic properties that allow the action potential to propagate along the surface of a membrane and also provide the basis for the integrative abilities of a membrane.

The voltage changes associated with electrotonic properties are small and passive—their generation does not in any direct way involve voltage-gated channels; they are termed *local responses* or *local potentials* throughout this discussion. The most important characteristic of electrotonic properties and the local responses associated with them is that their influence cannot spread very far along a cable or membrane; activity in such systems decreases as it spreads from its point of origin. In fact, the great biological significance of the action potential is that it provides special mechanisms for overcoming the limitations of a passive, electrotonic cable and transmits information over long distances without decrement or deformation.

■ LOCAL RESPONSES, THRESHOLD, TRIGGER ZONE

Local Response and Threshold

All local responses have certain features in common. They are relatively small (usually a few millivolts), they can summate with one another, they are graded in size with the amount of stimulus applied to produce them, and, if they reach a sufficient amplitude, they give rise to an action potential. Virtually all the input to a nervous system and all the intercellular communication are done by means of the production of local responses. Local potentials occur as receptor potentials in sensory nerve terminals; they occur at the postsynaptic membrane as the result of the release of chemical transmitter from presynaptic nerves; and they occur at the muscle endplate as the result of the release of acetylcholine from motor nerve terminals. Small, restricted voltage changes can be produced by injection of current into neurons (Figure 4-1), and these responses are also classified as local potentials.

Recalling that membrane conductance is changed by alterations in membrane voltage, we can see that any local response (e.g., synaptic potential) can affect membrane voltage and thus alter the conductance of voltage-gated channels—even a small depolarization can cause some voltage-gated channels to open (see Figure 3-10). For example, ionic currents through synaptic channels change the membrane potential, and this in turn influences the voltage-dependent channels for Na^+ and K^+. A depolarizing local response, although small and independently generated, would nonetheless secondarily turn on g_{Na} to some degree and allow some inward flow of sodium current. This same depolarization would also increase g_K, and the result would be a concomitant small increase in the efflux of K^+ ions. At the same time, sodium inactivation would be turned on to a small degree, and chloride ions would passively enter the cell as a result of the decreased internal negativity. Thus, with such small depolarizations we have a discrete amount of inward sodium current being counter-balanced by the efflux of potassium, the influx of chloride, and inactivation. Unless the induced sodium influx is large enough and fast enough, the opposing (leak) currents will override this initial effect of a depolarizing electrotonic event and repolarize the cell toward the resting potential.

Large local responses may cause enough depolarization, however, that the induced voltage-gated inward sodium current may be just balanced by the other competing ionic movements. If, at this stage, just a few more sodium ions come in, the membrane will be depolarized a little more and the action potential will suddenly begin and the positive feedback cycle illustrated in Figure 3-3 will take over.

Thus there is some membrane potential, depolarized from the resting level, at which the explosive, regenerative action potential mechanism is triggered. This level of depolarization is called the *threshold* of the action potential and corresponds to the degree of depolarization that will allow the inward movement of sodium ions to supersede the opposing ionic currents (mainly efflux of potassium). The actual membrane potential value of threshold varies from cell to cell and usually ranges from 5 to 20 mV depolarized from rest. Threshold can only be determined by observation or direct testing, such as by passing enough depolarizing current into the cell to finally trigger a spike (as illustrated in Figure 4-1). The local response then is a *subthreshold* amount of depolarization associated with less than an adequate amount of turn-on of g_{Na} to trigger an action potential. Local responses can also be negative-going or hyperpolarizing.

■ **QUESTIONS** *(Answers at end of chapter)*

1. List five major features of local responses.

2. Local responses occur as natural phenomena and can be produced experimentally. What are the two classes of biologically produced local potentials and how can local potentials be induced electrically?

3. What is threshold?

4. In terms of absolute numbers of millivolts, is the membrane potential closer to threshold at the peak of the spike potential or at the peak of the afterhyperpolarization?

5. Local potentials are important in a nervous system because they are able to depolarize the membrane to threshold and thus induce an _____ _____ .

6. Many very important local potentials, however, have just the opposite capability; they function to move the membrane away from threshold. They must therefore _____ the membrane or, in other words, make it go in the _____ direction.

The Trigger Zone

An important corollary to an understanding of the concept of threshold is that most neurons have a specialized region of their surface that has a lower threshold for spike initiation than other parts of the cell. This region of uniquely low threshold is often called the *trigger zone* and is the site where action potentials are initially generated in the cell. The reason the trigger zone has a low threshold is that an especially high density of voltage-gated Na^+ channels is located there. The location of the trigger zone has significant implications for the way a cell responds to local responses and for how neurons establish a normal functional directionality for action potential propagation. This can best be appreciated by examining the trigger zone in the classically studied spinal motor neuron (= motoneuron) (Figure 4-2). The trigger zone (area of lowest threshold) in these cells is located at the region of the axon hillock–initial segment (of the axon). Local responses produced by synaptic inputs onto the dendrites and soma of the cell do not normally lead to action potential generation where they are

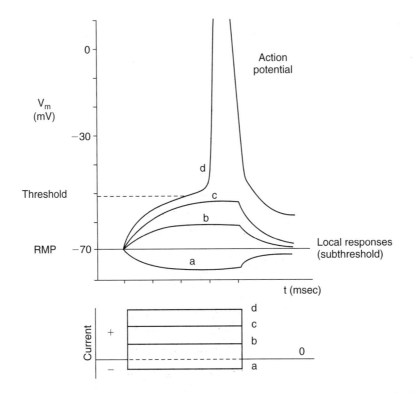

Figure 4-1 ■ Excitable cells can be brought to threshold by depolarizing currents. The lower part of the figure depicts small amounts of negative (*a*) or positive (*b-d*) current injected into a neuron by a microelectrode. Such current pulses induce small changes in membrane potential as shown above. These responses are called passive, electrotonic, or local responses. They rise on an exponential time scale to a plateau level proportional to the amount of current injected and then fall exponentially back to the resting potential with the current is turned off. If enough positive current is injected, the membrane may be depolarized enough to reach a threshold level at which an action potential is initiated (*d*). RMP, Resting membrane potential.

first produced because these parts of the cell have a high threshold (low excitability) resulting from a relative sparsity of voltage-gated Na⁺ channels. Local responses (synaptic potentials) instead spread decrementally over the surface of the soma-dendritic portions of the cell, summating with one another algebraically, until they eventually reach the trigger zone. If the local responses have not decayed too much, or if they have summed with enough other depolarizing inputs,

they may still produce an adequate amount of depolarization to bring the trigger zone to threshold and generate (trigger) an action potential. Thus the integrative properties of a neuron actually represent the way in which the passive properties of the soma-dendritic membrane allow local responses (synaptic potentials) to decrement and sum over the geometry of the surface.

When a spike is generated at the trigger zone, it will propagate away from this region as an all-

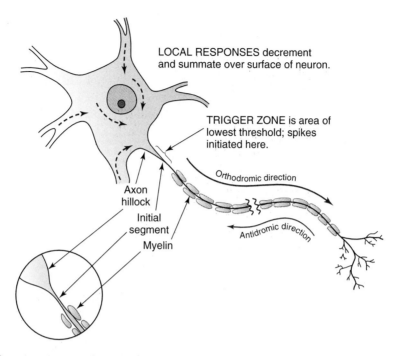

LOCAL RESPONSES decrement and summate over surface of neuron.

TRIGGER ZONE is area of lowest threshold; spikes initiated here.

Orthodromic direction

Antidromic direction

Axon hillock

Initial segment

Myelin

Figure 4-2 ■ The trigger zone of a spinal motoneuron. Like most nerve cells in the CNS, these neurons have a specific area on their membrane that has the lowest threshold for generating an action potential. This region of the cell is at the point where the axon leads off from the cell body. The cone-shaped taper of the soma is called the *axon hillock*. The initial segment of the axon is relatively thin, and then the axon diameter increases somewhat at the point where the first internode of myelin begins. There is an especially high density of voltage-gated sodium channels in the axon hillock–initial segment region, the trigger zone. When an action potential is initiated at the trigger zone, it then propagates down the axon as an orthodromic impulse to the terminals. An action potential that is artificially induced at some point on the axon can conduct toward the cell body, and this is called *antidromic propagation.*

or-nothing stereotyped electrical impulse. Thus the action potential propagates back over the surface of the soma and dendrites of the cell. It also propagates down the length of the axon of the motoneuron. The propagation of action potentials along the normal functional direction of impulse conduction of a cell is said to be *orthodromic* conduction (i.e., the normal direction). Thus for motoneurons the orthodromic direction of propagation is from the trigger zone

at the base of the axon in the central nervous system (CNS) outward toward the peripheral target organ. The motoneuron situation may be contrasted with that of a primary sensory neuron whose cell body is located in a dorsal root ganglion near the spinal cord and whose sensory axon is located in the periphery in association with some sense organ, for example, a touch corpuscle. The trigger zone (or region of lowest functional threshold) for this sensory cell is at the end of its axon where it is associated with the receptor. Again, this region has a high density of voltage-gated Na^+ channels (see Figure 4-13). Appropriate stimulation of the receptor will lead to a local response in the sensory axon terminal that can depolarize the ending to threshold. The spike generated here then propagates *orthodromically* from the periphery toward the CNS carrying sensory information. Note that the orthodromic direction is opposite for the motoneuron and the sensory cell.

Finally, a peripheral nerve can be stimulated experimentally with electrodes to test for effects of nerve stimulation. Action potentials can be generated almost anywhere along an axon with such artificial stimulation, and the spikes will propagate away, in both directions, from the point of initiation. Stimulation of the peripheral axon of a motoneuron will produce spikes that propagate toward the CNS, in the direction opposite to the natural flow of impulse traffic. The "backward" propagation is termed the *antidromic* direction and can provide important experimental information. For example, (1) since spikes can travel in either direction along an axon, the membrane properties that underlie action potential production are not oriented or designed in any directionally sensitive manner; and (2) if a nerve cell was penetrated in the spinal cord with a microelectrode to determine if it was a motoneuron, the spinal nerve could be stimulated from that segment of the cord to see whether antidromic action potentials could be produced in the cell.

■ QUESTIONS *(Answers at end of the chapter)*

7. The anatomical-physiological region of a neuron that has the lowest threshold is called the _____ _____ .

8. The direction along which action potentials travel during normal neurobiological

activity is called the _____ direction.

9. When action potentials propagate in the direction opposite to their normal conduction direction, the cell is said to conduct the impulses in the _____ _____ direction.

■ EXCITABILITY

The term *excitability* in a general sense means how readily one can induce an action potential in a nerve. If a neuron is very excitable, it is easily stimulated to produce an action potential and is said to have a low threshold. In a more strict sense, excitability is defined as the "reciprocal of threshold," i.e., as the threshold increases (becomes more difficult to attain), the excitability decreases. Or as threshold decreases, excitability increases.

Changes in Excitability of the Nerve Membrane during the Action Potential

During the course of an action potential the nerve membrane passes through several stages of excitability (Figure 4-3). The membrane is inexcitable for the duration of the spike potential. An action potential cannot be elicited at this time by a second stimulus of any amplitude, and the membrane is said to be *absolutely refractory*. The membrane then passes into a *relatively refractory* period that coincides with the last part of repolarization. Throughout this period the threshold is increased, and the amplitude of an evoked action potential is reduced. Finally, coexistent with the after-hyperpolarization is a period of reduced excitability, the *subnormal period*. The refractoriness of the membrane is due to a combination of the inactivation of sodium channels and the increased potassium conductance. The after-hyperpolarization, caused by the prolonged increase in the potassium conductance, accounts for the subnormal period.

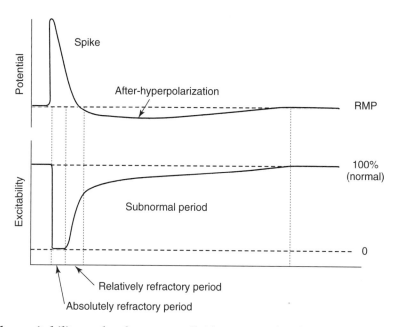

Figure 4-3 ■ **The excitability cycle of a nerve cell. The ease with which an action potential can be initiated, or induced, is referred to as a neuron's *excitability level*. The level of excitability is plotted on an arbitrary scale beneath a drawing of a typical action potential. After an action potential is begun and until the peak of the spike is over, the cell is said to be absolutely refractory—zero excitability (or maximum threshold). During this time another spike cannot be generated. In the late part of the repolarization phase the excitability increases. It is somewhat easier to generate another action potential during this period, but the spike will be abnormally small. During the period of the after-hyperpolarization, excitability is subnormal but gradually increases until it returns to its normal (100%) level. Threshold is elevated during the subnormal period, but adequate (increased) stimulation can produce a relatively normal action potential. *RMP,* Resting membrane potential.**

■ **QUESTIONS** *(Answers at end of chapter)*

10. What is meant by an increase in threshold? What relationship does excitability have to threshold?

11. What two factors account for the absolutely refractory period? Obviously, if the absolutely refractory period were longer in duration, the number of spikes per second would decrease ... Right?

12. Would the functional effect of hyperpolarizing a cell by injecting current be equivalent to the subnormal period?

Accommodation

If a subthreshold depolarizing current pulse or a slowly rising depolarizing pulse is applied to a nerve membrane, there will be an initial period of hyper-excitability caused by the partial depolarization, followed by a phase of decreased

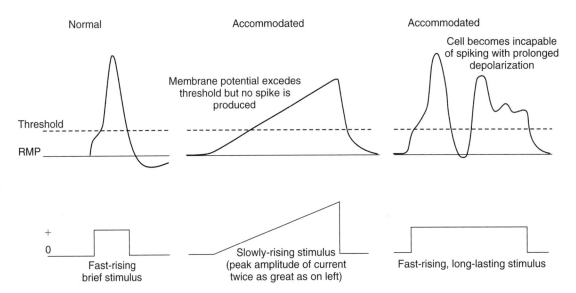

Figure 4-4 ■ Accommodation. *Left,* The normal case shows that a typical square wave of positive current *(lower trace)* lasting a few milliseconds depolarizes a nerve cell *(upper trace)* to threshold and a spike is generated. *Middle,* A depolarizing current that is given slowly enough, even though its peak value is much higher than a brief exciting current, can depolarize a neuron and move the membrane beyond threshold and still never generate an action potential. The cell is said to be accommodated. *Right,* Neurons can also be accommodated (made inexcitable) by a stimulating current pulse that initially produced spikes but with long application renders the cell incapable of further activity. *RMP,* Resting membrane potential.

excitability (increased threshold). In the case of electrical excitation (Figure 4-4), this means that a current is effective when it is applied initially but loses its effect during its continued passage. A current of slowly rising strength may not set up an impulse, even though it may rise gradually to an intensity many times greater than that at which a quickly rising square pulse is effective. This decline in excitability with prolonged depolarization is termed *accommodation,* and two membrane mechanisms are responsible for it: (1) inactivation of the sodium conductance and (2) increase in potassium conductance.

■ **QUESTIONS** *(Answers at end of the chapter)*

13. An amount of current five times greater

than the usual amount necessary to reach threshold is applied in such a manner as to avoid producing an action potential. What is this phenomenon called?

14. Sodium inactivation and increased potassium conductance account for the repolarization phase of the spike potential. These same two processes also account for the important passive membrane property just described in question 13. Name this process again, and watch the spelling this time.

15. How might one manipulate the extracellular

potassium concentration to render a cell inexcitable?

■ PASSIVE (ELECTROTONIC) PROPERTIES OF THE MEMBRANE

Electrical Elements of the Membrane

To this point the movements of ions and the forces that control these movements primarily have been considered in a straightforward chemical sense. To develop an understanding of the manner in which local responses spread and action potentials propagate along membranes, the membrane must be considered from an electrical model point of view.

The membrane of excitable cells separates the cytoplasm and extracellular fluids that contain dissolved ions experiencing the forces of electrical and concentration gradients. An ionic current (electrical current) in this system may be defined as the migration of ions down either an electrical field gradient or a concentration gradient. The imposed electrical field in this situation is the membrane potential. For example, sodium ions are "stored" as potential energy in a region of positivity (the outside of the membrane is about +70 mV relative to the inside), and this potential energy will be converted to the kinetic energy of movement of sodium inward whenever these ions are allowed to pass through the membrane.

Relatively speaking, the salty axoplasm and extracellular fluids are fairly good conductors of electrical currents. Over a unit length of axon, one centimeter long, the axoplasm has a resistance of around 30 ohms (Ω), and the surrounding extracellular fluid has a resistance of about 20 Ω. Compared with a copper wire, these solutions are poor conductors; however, the solutions are very good conductors compared with the membrane. The membrane behaves like an insulator and has a high electrical resistance—many times greater than that of its surrounding liquid media. The dimensions that are conventionally given to the membrane resistance are $\Omega \times cm^2$, and this value

is termed the *specific resistance* (R_m) of the membrane. The values of R_m may range from less than 1000 to near 10,000 Ωcm^2, depending on the surface area of the neuron and its characteristic response to applied currents. Values for R_m require knowledge of the entire surface area of a neuron (or treatment of the cell as a perfect sphere or closed cylinder so that surface area can be calculated from knowledge of the radius). This discussion is concerned with the movement of current across limited segments of membrane. Values for membrane resistance and longitudinal resistance of fluids that occur over 1-cm segments (unit length) of membrane will be adopted. This will provide a convenient means of describing the movements of local responses along a cylinder of axon or a dendrite. For the unit length of membrane, r_m will be used for membrane resistance in units of Ω-cm, and r_i and r_o for the resistance of axoplasm and extracellular fluid, respectively, in units of Ω/cm.

As introduced in Chapter 3, an expression that describes the relationship between resistance, electrical current, and electrical potential is Ohm's law:

$$V = IR$$

where
V = electrical potential
I = current
R = resistance

This equation describes the movement of ionic currents across the resistant membrane or down the axoplasm under the influence of an electrical field gradient. It should be clear that, under the influence of the same magnitude of electrical gradient, proportionately more current will flow over low-resistance pathways (fluids) than through high-resistance pathways (the membrane).

A material with high resistivity, such as this

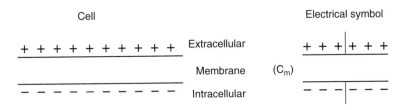

Figure 4-5 ■ The membrane has properties of a capacitor. *Left,* **A membrane with stored positive charge on its outer surface and stored negative charge on its cytoplasmic surface. This arrangement can be seen as a capacitor in an electrical circuit** *(right).* **The lipid membrane is a dialectric, and the stored charges can be thought of as sodium ions (+) on the outside and fixed anionic charges (–) on the intracellular membrane surface.**

membrane, is termed a *dielectric* or *insulator*. If a dielectric separates two electrically conductive materials, at different electrical potentials, charged particles within the conductors will migrate toward and are stored at the conductor-dielectric interface. These particles are attempting to lose potential energy by crossing the dielectric, but their movements are impeded by the dielectric's insulating characteristics. As the charged particles move to the conductor-dielectric interface, an electrical field begins to develop across the dielectric. Potential energy in the form of an electrical potential difference is stored on the dielectric. The electrical property of a dielectric material to store charges in this manner is termed *capacitance* (C). An electrical device consisting of two conductors, separated by a dielectric, is termed a *capacitor*. The unit of capacitance is the farad (F), and the capacitance of most membranes (C_m) is around 1 pF/cm^2. For a unit length of membrane the capacitance is written as c_m with units of F/cm.

The formula for determining capacitance is:

$$C = Q/V$$

where the storage capability, or capacitance, is equal to charge (Q) divided by voltage (V). The greater the capacitance, the more electrical charge that can be held across a dielectric with an applied voltage.

The membrane can be visualized as a capacitor (Figure 4-5), represented mainly by the bilayer of nonconductive membrane phospholipids. It has a very high resistance and is separating two highly conductive fluids, the cytoplasm and the extracellular fluid. Membrane voltage can be considered as stored electrical potential—the external positive charges (mainly sodium ions) on one surface of the membrane-capacitor and the internal negative charges (mainly organic anions [A$^-$]) on the inner face of the membrane-capacitor.

The nerve membrane has both electrical resistivity and capacitance. It behaves as a "leaky" capacitor, i.e., the capacitance of the membrane will be discharged through the resistive component of the membrane. The resistive pathways through the membrane are represented by the resting, leak channels that permit passive transmembrane ion flow when V_m is altered. In other words, while the membrane behaves as a capacitor (separates and stores charge across itself), it can also allow current (or charge) to move across it (through its resistive elements, channels). An electrical analog of a segment of a nerve membrane would consist of a resistor (R) and a capacitor (C) arranged in parallel, as shown in Figure 4-6. Such an arrangement is called an *RC circuit.*

■ **QUESTIONS** *(Answers at end of chapter)*

16. The highly structured, mostly lipid cell

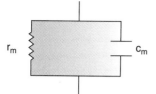

Where: c_m = membrane capacitance

r_m = membrane resistance

Figure 4-6 ■ Components of an RC circuit. A membrane acts like a resistor and a capacitor arranged in parallel, where c_m represents the stored charge on the membrane and r_m represents the passive leak (mainly K^+) channels through the membrane.

membrane has characteristics of a capacitor (i.e., it can store charge on its surfaces and maintains a voltage across itself). In addition, there are channels through the membrane that allow ionic current to move through the membrane. Thus the membrane acts like a resistor. The membrane capacitance (c_m) and resistance (r_m) are arranged, effectively, in series or in parallel? Electrically, this arrangement is referred to as an _____ circuit.

17. As the cross-sectional area of a wire increases, what happens to its resistance?

18. What is the practical application to passive membrane properties of the relationships of current, resistance, and voltage in Ohm's law?

19. Explain C = Q/V.

Resistor-Capacitor Circuit Characteristics

RC circuits (and the membrane) have electrical characteristics that result in allowing current to flow through them only on an *exponential time scale*. Figure 4-7 shows the way in which current flows through the membrane with a portion of membrane with an RC circuit superimposed over it. Current can flow through the membrane in two ways: as resistive current and as capacitative current.

Resistive current occurs as ions move through passive, non–voltage-sensitive (leak) channels in the membrane—symbolically, through the resistive element (r_m) of the RC circuit. Current (I_{ion}) moving through the resistor (r_m) will, by Ohm's law (IR = V), result in a change in the membrane voltage (V_m). Resistive current involves the actual physical transfer of an ion through the membrane, a transmembrane flow of ionic current, mainly occurring through the open K^+ channels that account for resting potassium conductance. This current flow is shown in Figure 4-7 as the outward movement of K^+ ions through the membrane (lumped leak channel) resistance r_m on the left of the RC circuit.

Capacitative current involves a net flow of current across the membrane—a change in charge stored across it—but does not require a transfer of an ion through the membrane. Capacitative current flow occurs when, for example, one of the anionic charges (A^-) inside the cell is neutralized, or cancelled, by some internal cation. This internal negative charge no longer attracts a positive charge on the opposite side of the membrane capacitor, and thus a sodium ion, for example, would be free to flow away from the surface of the cell. A true flow of current from inside to outside could be recorded, but no ions would pass through the membrane, only up to its inner surface and away from its outer surface. Note also that by reducing the amount of charge (Q) held

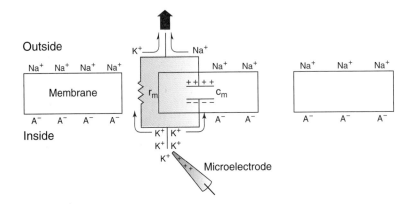

Figure 4-7 ■ Current flow throught the RC network of the membrane. Positive current is injected into this cell with the glass pipette electrode. The injected current repels intracellular K⁺ ions that move to the inner surface of the membrane. There, as symbolized by the two arms of the RC circuit, K⁺ ions may neutralize the fixed anionic charge (A⁻) of the capacitance (c$_m$, right arm of the circuit) or may move through the resistance (r$_m$) of the leaky membrane channels (left arm of the circuit drawn in a space representing a hydrophilic channel) to pass out of the cell.

across the membrane by its capacitance (C), which remains constant, the voltage across the membrane has been also reduced. (Recall that C = Q/V, and since C is constant, when Q goes down, so must V).

Thus, when a positive current is applied to the inside of the cell, as shown by the pipette electrode in Figure 4-7, the positive source will repel other nearby positive ions. These would be mostly potassium ions (K⁺), since they are by far the most numerous and most mobile of intracellular cations. The K⁺ ions will be driven toward the inner surface of the membrane and will begin to interact with the RC circuit there. At first, most of them are involved in discharging or neutralizing the capacitance by canceling out the negative charges (A⁻) near the membrane. This will then free up Na⁺ ions on the outer surface. Capacitative current flows, the charge on c$_m$ is reduced; the membrane voltage begins to be reduced from its original high negative resting value toward a more positive value and the cell starts to be depolarized.

Some K⁺ ions are also flowing away from the applied positive source and are moving through the resistive arm of the RC circuit. These ions are flowing through the membrane out of the cell (at rest the membrane is quite permeable to potassium). As the capacitance is discharged and the voltage is reduced (made less negative), more potassium flows out through the membrane under the new driving force (i.e., K⁺ will be driven away by the increased intracellular positivity) until a steady state is reached, at which time the capacitance has been discharged and the voltage has reached some new steady value. *The potassium is leaving the cell at the same rate that the positive current is being applied by the electrode.* This new voltage, or potential, level will remain constant until the current is turned off. Figure 4-8 illustrates the major feature of the voltage change: *it occurs on an exponential time scale.* Despite the fact that the current was applied in a fast step pulse (square pulse), the membrane "took time" to respond to this application of current. Because of the RC character-

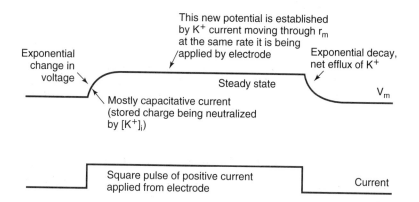

Figure 4-8 ▪ The application of a small (subthreshold) amount of positive current (square wave below) in a neuron produces a voltage change that begins and ends with a change in transmembrane potential that occurs on an exponential time scale. The initial depolarization represents the change in V_m that proceeds by the simultaneous occurrence of neutralization of capacitative charge and outward K^+ movement through r_m. A new steady-state V_m is reached when the capacitative current flow is completed (the amount of new charge, Q, added by the electrode has had time to bring V_m to a new level), and K^+ ions are now leaving the cell through r_m at the same rate they are being injected by the electrode. When we turn off the injected current, K^+ ions will continue to leave the cell (the cell is highly permeable to K^+ ions at rest and the membrane potential has been displaced away from E_K—see Figure 2-3), carrying away positive charge and simultaneously "uncovering" internal anionic charges. The fall back to the original resting potential is established, in other words, by a net outward movement of positivity through the RC circuit.

istics of the passive membrane, all subthreshold voltage changes (i.e., all local or electrotonic responses) occur exponentially. This process is described in more detail in the next section. These same properties also prohibit local responses from traveling far over the surface of the membrane.

▪ **QUESTIONS** *(Answers at end of chapter)*

20. Explain (in words) the difference between capacitative and resistive currents at the membrane.

21. Is the rate at which a capacitor will lose or gain charge linear or exponential? Will the voltage across the capacitor change at the same rate?

Fate of Local Responses over the Space of the Membrane and Time

The area of the membrane is represented repeatedly by many RC circuits arranged in parallel throughout the entire surface of a cell. Represented in Figure 4-9 is an edge-on view of a short length of membrane with several RC circuits joining the intracellular and extracellular fluids. Each $r_m c_m$ circuit represents the lumped resistance and capacitance of a one-cm unit-length of axon. The RC circuits are tied together inside and outside by series resistances assigned, respectively, to the intracellular (r_i) and extracellular fluids (r_o). The behavior of local responses as they spread over such a surface (or along a length) of membrane is examined by applying a source of current from a battery, whose positive

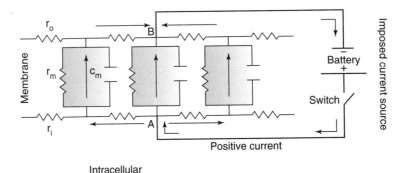

Figure 4-9 ■ **Passive electrical circuit over a segment of membrame. Three parallel RC circuits are shown in a side-on view of a small stretch of membrane representing a length of dendrite or axon cylinder. Any longitudinal currents running inside the cylinder are seen to pass through the intracellular resistance, r_i. Extracellular currents run through r_o. The text describes the movement of positive current through this circuit when we artificially apply a square pulse of positive current to the inside of the cell at point A. The injection system is shown as a simple battery. Generally, the positive current carried into the cell will move away from point A, carried by the abundant and mobile K^+ ions inside. These ions can move longitudinally through r_i or can participate as transmembrane currents via the RC circuits repeated in the membrane. To complete the circuit, positive current will leave the area outside the membrane at point B.**

pole is connected to the inside of the cell at point A and whose negative pole is attached to a point (B) in the extracellular fluid. When the switch is closed, a constant flow of positive current will be applied to the inside of the cell until the switch is opened. This uniform method of stimulation is convenient for analysis, but recall that the types of natural stimuli a cell receives, such as synaptic inputs, are not so regularly shaped, although they are handled in the same way by the circuitry.

When the switch is closed, the electrode begins to inject positive charges into the cell (*point A,* Figure 4-9). This will drive potassium ions, which are positively charged, away from the electrode and toward the membrane. Part of this potassium current could flow through the capacitive elements of the membrane and

part through the resistive elements. The observed voltage change across the membrane occurs slowly in response to an abruptly applied current because time is required for the flow of charges (potassium ion current) to alter the amount of charge on the capacitor and thus the voltage across it. At the instant the switch is closed, all the potassium current is involved in neutralizing the capacitative charge; there is no current through the resistive elements because the potential across the resistive elements and capacitative elements is the same.* As time passes, more and more potassium ions move to the membrane inner surface to neutralize the fixed negative charges and thus reduce the transmembrane potential. As the membrane potential changes, some current is then diverted to the resistive element, and the rate of discharging the capacitor is correspondingly decreased. This process continues—more and more current flows through the resistance of the membrane and less and less through the capacitance—until finally all the current is flowing through the resistance. At this point the capacitative current changes are over, and a new steady-state voltage has been induced in the cell.

If the membrane had a low capacitance, relatively few potassium ions would be used up in discharging the capacitance and establishing a voltage change across the resistance of the membrane. If, on the other hand, the membrane had a high capacitance, then more potassium ions would be used up in neutralizing the capacitative charge and setting up a voltage change. This process of potassium either neutralizing the capacitance or eventually crossing the membrane as a transmembrane current through a resistor will continue until the voltage across the capacitor is sufficient to drive potassium ions out of the membrane at exactly the same rate positive charges are being delivered from the electrode. The rate at which the steady state voltage level is achieved will be influenced by both the resistance and the capacitance of the membrane. An increase in either r_m or c_m tends to slow the rate of change. If r_m is increased, potassium can less readily move

---

*By analyzing this statement, we have an opportunity to look at the Ohm's relationship from another perspective. At the resting potential, a steady-state condition very near E_K, there is virtually no net ionic current across the membrane. No K^+ current (I) is moving through r_m because V_m is near E_K and the electrical and concentration gradients on potassium are balanced. Thus, at rest, V_m is constant, r_m is constant, so I (transmembrane current) is constant: $I = V/R$. As long as V_m and r_m are unchanged, there can be no net flow of ions across the membrane. When the current is artificially injected into the cell with the electrode, the charge (Q) on the membrane is reduced; this leads to a reduction in membrane potential. Now, since V_m has changed (let us say it was reduced from –70 to –65 mV), a current flow must be present. Thus potassium ions move out of the cell through r_m, as they should, since the negativity holding them inside at rest has been reduced.

through the membrane to change V_m. If c_m is large, a larger amount of current (and time) will be used up in discharging the capacitance and changing V_m. This exponential process can be characterized by a single parameter for varying sizes of current pulse. Formally, the following equation can describe the rising phase of the potential change:

$$V_t = V_o(1 - e^{-t/\tau})$$

where
V_t = Change in potential with respect to time
V_o = Initial value of membrane potential
e = Base for natural logarithms (= approx. 2.7, or 3)
τ = Membrane time constant

This time constant is equal to the product of the membrane resistance and the membrane capacitance ($\tau = r_m c_m$). If we waited for a time equal to the time constant (i.e., let t = τ) to look at the amplitude of a voltage change, then the voltage at that time (V_t) would equal the original voltage (V_o) times $(1-e^{-1})$, or $(1-1/e) = (1 - \sim1/3)$, or approximately 2/3 (63%) of the maximum change. The *time constant* (τ) is the time for any potential to rise to 2/e (~ 2/3 or 63%) of its final value or to fall to 1/e (~1/3 or 37%) of its initial value (where $V_t = V_o e^{-t/\tau}$) (Figure 4-10). The time it takes for any passive (subthreshold) response in the same cell to rise to 2/e of its final size or drop to 1/e of its original size will be constant. On the other hand, the time it takes for responses of the same size in two *different* cells to reach 1/e or 2/e of their final size will be different if c_m or r_m in the two cells is different.

When capacitances are placed in parallel, they increase the total capacitance. Consequently, as potentials spread farther away from the point at which the potential is being applied, the apparent capacitance will get larger and larger and the responses become progressively smaller and more distorted. The effect of having a capaci-

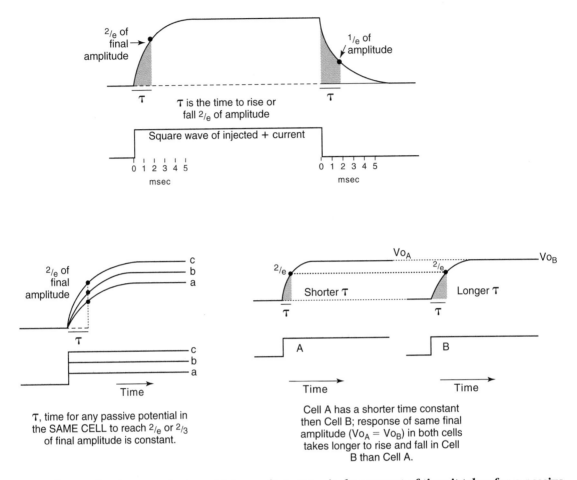

Figure 4-10 ■ The time constant τ, which equals $c_m \times r_m$, is the amount of time it takes for a passive voltage change to get 2/e of the way through its change. The time constant is the same for all responses in the same cell *(lower left)* but may be different in two different cells *(lower right),* even for voltage changes of the same amplitude.

tance in parallel with a membrane resistance is to reduce the height of a potential and to slow down its rate of change.

The spread of ionic current through the circuit of Figure 4-9 can be examined from the point of view of the resistive current flow (i.e., how the steady-state current is distributed through r_m, r_o and r_i after the capacitative discharging is

complete). When the switch is closed, the applied positive current will repel cations (mainly K^+) from region A, and these ions could flow either through r_m or along r_i. However, the membrane is a good insulator; in other words, it hinders the flow of current or ions. This means that potassium ions that come up against the membrane will not be able to leave immediately but will

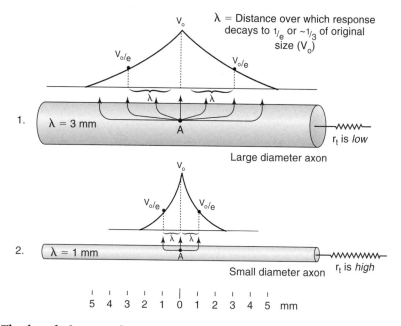

Figure 4-11 ■ The length (or space) constant, λ, is obtained as the square root of $r_m/(r_i + r_o)$. It represents how far a passive change in V_m will spread before it decreases to 1/e of its initial size, V_o. The length constant is longer in larger-diameter axons *(1)* as compared to small-diameter axons *(2)*.

accumulate and spread laterally down the low-resistance pathway (r_l). A transmembrane voltage change will occur only at the region where potassium ions are crossing the membrane (i.e., I_K through r_m causes a change in V_m). The degree of voltage change is directly proportional to the amount of current passing through the membrane (Figure 4-11). The potential will spread further if the membrane resistance is high or if the lateral (longitudinal) resistance, r_i, is low. Potassium ions will move further down the membrane's inner surface before they cross the membrane to change potential. If the membrane resistance were low, potassium could leave the cell without spreading so far along under the membrane, and the transmembrane voltage change would be restricted to a small area of membrane. In the external circuit, once the current has been carried across the membrane, other ions will carry the charges toward the negative pole, or cathode (chloride ions will tend to move away from the negative pole, and sodium ions will tend to move toward it).

If the fiber is very small in diameter, there will be fewer ions present in the axoplasm to carry current in any one cross-sectional area. Therefore there will be a higher r_i resistance and a steeper longitudinal fall of voltage (lateral current flow will be restricted) (see axon *2* in Figure 4-11). Exactly the same applies to the effect of external resistance. The higher r_o, the more drastically the spread of potential will be curtailed. The movement of potassium ions, caused by injecting positive charges, makes some of them leave the leaky membrane at the point of application of the current pulse; in the neighboring region of the membrane, fewer potassium ions have accumulated and therefore fewer leak out, and so on all the way along the nerve. The number of potassium ions leaving a unit area of membrane is going to vary in an exponential manner with the distance away from the current-passing electrode. This means that the transmembrane voltage change will decay, or decrease, exponentially from the site of initiation (see *point A* in Figure 4-11, axon *1*) over the surface of the membrane.

One characteristic of this exponential function is that no matter what the size of the voltage change at the initiation site, its amplitude will decrease to l/e (~1/3 or 37%) of the original size over a certain distance. The distance over which a potential falls to 1/e of its original size is a characteristic length for a particular nerve or muscle fiber and is known as the *length* or *space* constant, λ (see Figure 4-11). It will increase with increased membrane resistance, and it will decrease with an increased internal or external resistance. In fact, $\lambda = \sqrt{r_m/(r_i+r_o)}$. It has the dimensions of length (precisely, centimeters: $\sqrt{\Omega cm/\Omega/cm} = \sqrt{cm^2} = cm$), and although it may be as large as 1 mm in a muscle, it will be much less in a small nerve fiber (perhaps only a few microns). The formal equation for computing the change in V_m over a distance "x" is

$$V_x = V_o\, e^{-x/\lambda}$$

If one moves a distance x that is equal to λ (or $\sqrt{r_m/(r_i+r_o)}$) from the site of an induced subthreshold voltage change (V_o), then the size of the potential at that distance will be V_o/e, or about 37% of the original potential.

The composition of the cytoplasm does not vary from one axon or dendrite to another. What does vary is the *diameter* of the process and the number of ions available for carrying current. Thus the effective internal resistance, r_i, is greater in small-diameter fibers than in large ones, and, consequently, the length constant is smaller in small fibers than in large ones. The distance over which a subthreshold voltage change is reduced to 1/e of its original size will be shorter in small-diameter axons and dendrites (such potentials will "die out" sooner or be less effective). Under most conditions, the external resistance r_o remains small and constant and is not critical.

▪ QUESTIONS   *(Answers at end of chapter)*

22. What is the formula for calculating the time constant, τ? What are the units for this constant?

23. Explain in words why an increase in either r_m or c_m could make the time constant longer.

24. When a local response has been reduced in amplitude by 1/e of its original size, the distance over which that response has traveled (x) can be calculated by the formula _____. This value is called the _____.

25. What is the most common intracellular small inorganic cation? Now, what does diameter have to do with r_i?

26. Neuron "A" has a time constant of 1 msec, while neuron "B" has a time constant of 2 msec. Each cell has the same resting potential, and this membrane potential is displaced in each cell by a brief injection of depolarizing (subthreshold) current. In which cell will the membrane potential most rapidly return to the resting level?

The passive electrical properties of the membrane make it impossible for local potentials to propagate over large distances. They decline sharply over distances of less than a millimeter, and their time course also becomes blurred. Although they cannot propagate, they are, how-

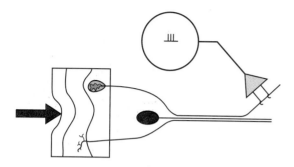

Figure 4-12 ■ Recording discharges from a single afferent fiber. A group of nerve fibers is shown innervating several types of receptor organs in the skin. A single axon has been dissected from the nerve bundle so that afferent impulses from just one kind of sensory receptor can be recorded on an oscilloscope (represented as circle attached to amplifier). The stimulus is symbolized by the arrow indenting the skin. An adequate stimulus will generate a train of action potentials (*upward lines* on the oscilloscope trace).

ever, extremely important in the nervous system because they can sum algebraically with one another over the soma-dendritic surface and change membrane potential relative to threshold. In addition, they are important for the normal propagation of the action potential. One great family of local responses include synaptic potentials, which are discussed in Chapters 6 and 7. Another example of a family of naturally occurring local responses are the subthreshold potentials associated with sensory receptors. These are discussed briefly here.

Local Responses at Sensory Endings

A subset of neurons in any nervous system is specialized to transduce sensory stimuli, such as touch or pressure, temperature, pain, light, sound, and so on, that arrive from the environment or from within the body. These sensory neurons have a peripheral axon that ends in the skin, muscle, viscera or more specialized sense organs

(such as the eye and inner ear). The terminals of these peripheral axons, called *receptor or sensory endings*, have the task of converting stimuli, such as mechanical energy, into action potentials that can propagate from the periphery to the central nervous system to relay meaningful information about the stimuli. (Sensory axons are also called *afferent* axons, or fibers, because their normal [orthodromic] direction of action potential propagation is toward the CNS. Motor axons are designated as *efferent* fibers, since they conduct orthodromically away from the CNS to peripheral muscles.) Certain of these mechano-sensitive afferent axons illustrate the role of local potentials in inducing action potentials. The activity in single afferent fibers can be recorded from particular kinds of mechanosensory endings (Figure 4-12). Appropriate stimulation, such as pressure or mechanical distortion in the region of the ending, will result in a train of action potentials in the axon. Under favorable conditions, most recently using patch-clamp recording from the membrane of the axon terminal in certain model systems, it is possible to record *receptor potentials* from the region of the sensory receptor or even to record activity from single mechanosensitive channels. A receptor potential is a graded, subthreshold depolarization—a local response—whose amplitude depends on the strength of the applied stimulus (Figure 4-13). The receptor potential may be large enough to reach threshold for evoking an action potential in the afferent axon, depending on the intensity of the stimulus.

The mechanism by which receptor potentials are produced in mechanoreceptors involves mechanical deformation of the axon terminal. Although the exact structural basis for the event is not certain, it is likely that the deformation works by disturbance of the lipid bilayer and associated cytoskeletal proteins. What is now clear is that these micromovements cause the opening of specialized channels in the terminal

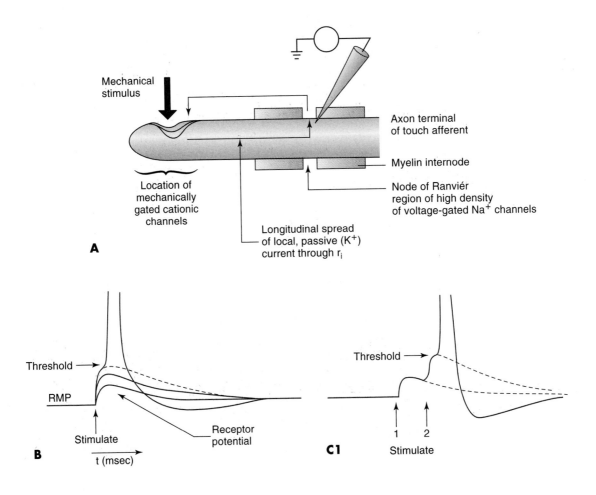

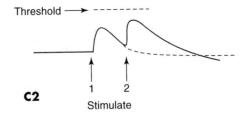

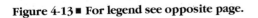

Figure 4-13 ■ For legend see opposite page.

Figure 4-13 ■ Responses produced by mechanical distortion of touch receptors are examples of local responses. A, Schematic drawing of the axon terminal of a sensory nerve fiber specialized to detect touch (mechanical indentation of the skin). The myelin sheath of the axon stops a short distance from the bare terminal. The terminal membrane has mechanosensitive channels that open when the membrane is distorted as by pressure to the skin surface, indicated by the large arrow where three successively stronger stimuli are applied. Voltage-gated Na^+ channels are densely packed in the axon membrane at the first node of Ranviér between the first two myelin internodes. A microelectrode is used to record changes in membrane potential in the terminal region. B, A mild touch to the skin (the first stimulus drawn in A) causes a shallow indentation of the terminal membrane and opens a few mechanosensitive channels that produce a small depolarizing response called a *receptor potential*. Stronger mechanical stimulation causes a larger receptor potential. The depolarization at the terminal, produced by net influx of cations through the mechanosensitive channels, spreads as a wave of positivity along the axon membrane toward its myelinated portion. The depolarizing longitudinal electrotonic current carried by $[K^+]_i$ is indicated by the arrow inside the axon in A (see Figure 4-9). Because of the passive RC circuitry of the membrane, the receptor potential decrements as it moves along the axon membrane. If a stimulus is large enough, or if the length constant of the membrane is long enough so that the receptor potential does not decrement too much, then the receptor potential will still be of adequate amplitude to depolarize the area of membrane at the node, where Na^+ channels are located, to reach threshold for an action potential (*top* trace in B). C demonstrates how two receptor potentials can sum together and how the time constant can influence integration of such responses. In C1 a stimulus *(1)* is applied that causes a subthreshold receptor potential. A few milliseconds later the same stimulus is applied again *(2)*. The second receptor potential of the same amplitude as the first summates with the initial response and brings the membrane potential enough depolarized to reach threshold and start an action potential. Dotted line shows the full time course of the decay of the receptor potentials had they been allowed to proceed. C2 repeats the same experiment in a terminal with a shorter time constant, meaning that passive, local responses will decay faster than they would if produced in the axon in C1. Here, the same stimulus *(1)* produces a receptor potential of the same amplitude as the one in C1, but the response decays faster. If we repeat the stimulus *(2)* with the same delay as was used as the interstimulus interval in C1, the same-sized receptor potential is produced, but the total depolarization produced by the two summed responses is not enough to cause an action potential. The reason is that the first receptor potential decayed so rapidly that when the second response was added to the small amount of depolarization left in the decrementing first receptor potential, the peak of the second response could not reach threshold. *RMP,* Resting membrane potential.

---

membrane. Such mechanosensitive channels are part of a large family of related channels with prokaryotic ancestors. In general, the channels behave with discrete openings and closings (more openings with greater deformation or pressure) like other channels discussed, but these channels tend to have less ionic selectivity and higher unitary conductances. Most of the channels are permeable to a mix of cations, including Na^+, K^+ and Ca^{++} (these are typically called *cationic*

channels), but the dominant effect of channel opening is to cause a net increase in inward positive current (carried by Na^+ and Ca^{++}) based on the electrochemical gradients on these ions. Thus the rising (depolarizing) phase of a receptor potential is caused by an increased permeability to sodium ions in particular. Small deformations open a few channels, producing small inward Na^+ currents and small-amplitude depolarizations, while larger deformations open more channels and cause greater depolarizations. Each receptor potential increases the excitability of the ending by bringing the membrane potential nearer threshold, and large receptor potentials can reach threshold and generate an action potential. Action potentials can be generated in the region of the sensory terminal because nearby, usually at the first node of Ranviér in myelinated touch afferents, there is a high density of voltage-gated sodium channels. The depolarization caused by the receptor potential (essentially a brief pulse of positivity injected into the terminal not different from our injection of positivity at point A inside a nerve membrane in Figure 4-9) repels intracellular K^+ ions that move as local, electrotonic current away from the site of injection along the axon to depolarize the regions of the axon that contain the Na^+ channels. If the amount of spreading depolarization is large enough to open enough Na^+ channels, an action potential is generated.

The amplitude of the receptor potential will depend on the number of mechanically gated channels the deformation causes to open (Figure 4-13, B). Whatever the size of the receptor potential, channels remain open only a relatively short time and then close again. Thus the peak of the receptor potential is due to a net influx of positive current through specialized channels, but the decay of the receptor potential is carried out by the passive RC circuitry of the terminal membrane. How far and how rapidly the response spreads from the terminal is dependent on the passive properties of the membrane. If the length constant (λ) of the terminal membrane is relatively large, then a receptor potential may not decay too much by the time it spreads to the Na^+-channel-rich area of the axon to generate a spike. A receptor potential of the same initial size produced in a terminal with a shorter length constant could decrement too much to be adequate to bring the same nodal region to threshold. On the other hand, if a second receptor potential

were produced by a repeated touch at a short interval after the initial, subthreshold touch, then the second response could add algebraically to the first, and the summed response could be large enough to initiate an action potential (see Figure 4-13, $C1$). The time constant (τ) can play a role in this situation. If the terminal membrane has a relatively long time constant, meaning local potentials decay relatively slowly, then a second receptor potential would begin from a more depolarized level of V_m on the "tail" of the initial response as compared to the level of V_m at which it would start in a terminal with a shorter time constant where the decrementing first receptor potential had decayed more rapidly toward the resting potential (see Figure 4-13, $C2$).

Function of Local Responses

Local responses are passive, subthreshold potential changes in excitable cell membranes that can be produced at synapses (as explored later), at sensory endings (as examined here), or as "artificial" events produced by injected currents. Their behavior depends on the electrotonic, RC-circuit–like properties of membranes. Local potentials may be depolarizing or hyperpolarizing, are graded in amplitude, and can sum with one another algebraically. The local currents spreading from one origination point simply add with currents generated from some other point as they come together over the space of the membrane and in time, but all local potentials decay over time and along the membrane as they spread. Until and unless their summed amplitude reaches threshold, these responses just fade away. However, each depolarization (though passive in nature) is secondarily influencing g_{Na}, turning on this conductance proportionately with each depolarization. At the depolarized potential threshold, suddenly the independent and automatic conductance mechanisms for the action potential are activated. g_{Na} has been increased to a critical point, and now other, non-passive events with their own kinetics take over. The special voltage-gated Na^+ and K^+ channels have been opened. The membrane uses the stored potential energy of its sodium (E_{Na}) and potassium (E_K) batteries to superimpose the large active action potential over its passive components. The regenerative nature of the action potential overcomes the restrictive and passive characteristics of the membrane and now relays uniform impulses over its entire length. The way in which propagation occurs is the subject of Chapter 5.

■ POST-TEST

1. If the threshold of a nerve cell were 10 mV depolarized from the resting potential, would a local potential of 20 mV, produced 2 length constants away from the trigger zone, make the cell fire an action potential?

2. The length constant, λ, is known to be directly proportional to the square root of the fiber radius, y. Therefore another formula for computing the length constant would be:

$$\lambda = \sqrt{yR_m/(r_i + r_o)}$$

A nonmyelinated crustacean axon of 30 μ diameter (y = 15 x 10^{-4} cm) has a specific resistance, R_m, = 5,000 ohm-cm², and $r_i = r_o$ = 50 ohm-cm. Compute the length constant in millimeters.

3. We have always said in the past that when there was an outward potassium current, positive charges that were leaving the cell would consequently hyperpolarize the cell. Yet, we now say that outward potassium current through the RC network is associated with a depolarization of the cell. Explain.

4. If local responses can summate, what would happen to the membrane potential if equally sized depolarizing and hyperpolarizing local responses occurred simultaneously?

5. Using the circuit diagram of a membrane shown below, answer the questions about it using only the information shown on the diagram, assuming a normally-behaving membrane.
   (a) Is A inside or outside the cell?
   (b) Is the resistance GF in series or in parallel with resistance AH?
   (c) When positive current is injected with an electrode at point A and goes across the membrane, would you expect more or less current at E relative to D?
   (d) In a normal resting membrane, on which side of the c_m symbol would "+" be?
   (e) Would an increase in r_m cause more current to get from A to G?
   (f) What's the capacitance between F and H?

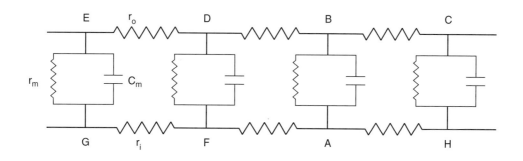

(g) During the earliest current flow (when c_m is being discharged) one possible current path would be *A* to *B* to *C.* What ion would most likely carry the current from *B* to *C?*

(h) Is r_m smaller than r_o?

(i) Could a potassium ion move from *A* to *B?* Symbolically, would it travel through r_m or c_m? If c_m were decreased, would K^+ ions get across the membrane sooner?

(j) With respect to transmembrane current, are the capacitors arranged in series or in parallel? Capacitors arranged in series can store more or less charge than capacitors in parallel?

(k) When current is injected at *A,* will current leave the membrane at *E* as fast as it leaves at *B?*

(l) A local potential induced at *A* would take longer to reach its peak and would decay more slowly if τ were larger. To achieve this, either _____ _____or _____ or both would have to be made larger. The response would move farther along the fiber if λ were increased. This would happen if _____ were larger or if _____ were smaller.

6. Depolarizing local responses act first to discharge some of the membrane capacitance, thus displacing the membrane potential in the positive direction and consequently allowing potassium to move out of the cell through the resistive current pathway of the system. If the total amount of depolarization is large enough, there is another ion waiting in the wings for its opportunity to get into the act, and it does. What is the mystery ion, and what has happened to allow it to get into the act (not to mention the cell)?

7. What is a receptor potential?

■ **REFERENCES AND ADDITIONAL READINGS**

Aidley DJ: *The physiology of excitable cells,* ed 4, Cambridge, 1998, Cambridge University Press.

French AS: Ion channels underlying transduction and adaptation in mechanoreceptors. In Urban L (ed): *Cellular mechanisms of sensory processing,* NATO ASI series, Heidelburg, 1993, Springer-Verlag.

Hamill OP, Martinac B: Molecular basis of mechanotransduction in living cells, *Physiol Rev* 81:685-740, 2001.

Hodgkin AL: The conduction of the nervous impulse, Springfield, Ill, 1964, Charles C Thomas.

Hodgkin AL, Rushton WAH: The electrical constants of a crustacean nerve fiber, *Proc R Soc Lond B Biol Sci* 133:444-479, 1946.

Jack JB, Noble D, Tsien RW: *Electric current flow in excitable cells,* Oxford, 1975, Oxford University Press.

Koester J, Siegelbaum SA: Local signalling: passive electrical properties of the neuron. In Kandel ER, Schwartz JH, Jessell TM (eds): *Principles of neural science,* ed 4, New York, 2000, McGraw-Hill, pp 140-149.

Nicholls JG, Martin AR, Wallace BG, et al: *From neuron to brain,* ed 4, Sunderland, Mass, 2001, Sinauer Assocoiates, pp 113-132.

Rall W: Core conductor theory and cable properties of neurons. In Kandel ER (ed): *Handbook of physiology: a critical, comprehensive presentation of physiological knowledge and concepts,* vol 1, Bethesda, Md, 1977, American Physiological Society, pp 39-97.

■ **ANSWERS**
Text Questions

1. They are relatively small; they are graded in size in proportion to stimulus intensity; they can summate with one another; they decrement over time and over the surface of the cell (i.e., they cannot spread very far); they can be negative- or positive-going in sign, and the latter may be large enough or can summate to depolarize the cell to threshold.

2. Local responses occur naturally as receptor

potentials in the endings of various sensory axons, and they are also represented by synaptic potentials that occur in nerve cells or in other postsynaptic elements such as muscle fibers. Experimentally, local responses are produced by injecting small amounts (subthreshold) of current into excitable cells. These small pulses perturb the passive electrical properties of the cell and allow one to examine the electrical characteristics of any biological membrane.

3. Threshold is a *level of membrane potential*, normally depolarized a few millivolts from the resting membrane potential (RMP), at which an action potential will be produced. It represents the membrane potential at which the inward sodium current exceeds the outward, counteracting potassium current.

4. Peak of the after-hyperpolarization.

5. Action potential.

6. Hyperpolarize; negative.

7. Trigger zone.

8. Orthodromic.

9. Antidromic.

10. An increase in threshold means functionally that a neuron becomes more difficult to excite (or made to fire action potentials); this most commonly occurs when the cell is hyperpolarized, the membrane potential then being further away from the threshold value. Sometimes the threshold value of membrane potential itself may also be altered, particularly by certain drugs or by cooling. Threshold is also elevated in the presensce of sodium inactivation because voltage-gated sodium channels cannot open. Excitability and threshold are inversely related.

11. Sodium inactivation and increased potassium conductance. Right.

12. No, not really. Although either current injection or after-hyperpolarization would put the membrane potential an equal distance away from threshold, leaving a similarly greater voltage change to be overcome to induce spiking, the latter situation would more effectively retard another spike because an increase in sodium conductance would have to be great enough not only to reach threshold but also to counteract the opposing potassium currents operating under the increased g_K during the subnormal period.

13. Accommodation.

14. Accommodation.

15. Recalling that the RMP is mostly dependent on resting potassium permeability, one can cause a change in RMP by altering $[K^+]_o$ (see Figure 2-4). Thus, if the extracellular K^+ concentration were increased by a factor of 2, the Nernst equation predicts that E_K would shift from about –75 mV to about –58 mV in squid axon. This 17 mV depolarization might well take the membrane potential beyond threshold and initially cause some action potentials. However, the depolarization would persist and the axon would become accommodated and effectively blocked.

16. Parallel; RC circuit.

17. Resistance goes down.

18. Ohm's law, an expression of the relationships between voltage, current, and resistance in a simple circuit, states that current moving through a resistor (IR) will result in a change in voltage (V). The application of this relationship to the passive membrane is that membrane potential, V_m, will change if ionic current (I) moves through the membrane resistance (r_m). For example, the resting potential will be altered if potassium ions move through the membrane, and the amount of voltage change will be proportional to how much current moves through and the magnitude of the membrane resistance. There are aspects of this phenomenon that must be carefully understood. First, this is a purely "passive" biological membrane whose resistance (r_m) is a fixed, stable value dependent on the number of passive, resting, or leak channels in a fixed length of membrane. This may be contrasted with the membrane resistance during an action potential, when, for unique reasons having to do with the special voltage-sensitive channels of the membrane, r_m actually changes and becomes very low, (i.e., the channels open up [resistance goes way down or conductance goes up]). Thus, for the case of the action potential, a big voltage change occurs because a lot of current can move across a very low resistance. For passive, subthreshold events, r_m is relatively high and does not permit much current to move and thus the voltage changes are small. Another important aspect of the Ohmic relationship is that in the passive resting state, the membrane potential is stable and in a steady state; currents do not suddenly move through the membrane "creating" voltages. The local potentials always represent the response of the system to some type of perturbation, which, as an "extrinsic" force, causes current to move. For example, the experimenter "adds" current to a cell by passing current (from an extrinsic voltage source) into the cell. Biologically, the passive cell is perturbed by, for example, receptor and synaptic potentials, which for our purposes may be thought of as brief applications of transmembrane current to which the cell responds with its passive circuitry. The more current (I) that is presented to the membrane resistance (r_m, which is constant), the more we will alter the transmembrane potential (V_m). Finally, it is important to note that the sign or direction (+ or –, depolarizing or hyperpolarizing) of the induced change in voltage is independent of the actual ohmic relationship. The positive or negative direction of the voltage change depends on which ionic currents flow across the membrane. If K^+ ions flow out of the cell, across r_m, then the net effect on V_m will be negative; if Na^+ ions come into the cell, V_m will move in the positive direction. If Cl^- ions move inward, the cell would become more negative. It is very important to understand, however, that the ions that do move across the membrane and cause V_m to change do so in response to an applied source of perturbation. Exactly which ion moves and in which direction depends on the polarity and magnitude of the extrinsic input; the induced ionic current movements always tend to restore the membrane to a steady-state, resting condition.

19. Opposite electrical charges (Q) can be stored on the two surfaces of a dielectric, and the application of these charges will create a potential difference (V) across the

dielectric. How well (or how much) charge can be separated or stored across the dielectric depends on a property of the dielectric called capacitance (C). The greater the capacitance or storage ability of the dielectric, the more charge it can effectively separate for a given potential difference across the dielectric (C = Q/V). In other words, dielectrics or capacitors with a very large capacitance can separate a large amount of charge at a given voltage. It will take longer to neutralize the stored charge on a large capacitor before the voltage will change. As with passive membrane resistance, r_m, membrane capacitance, c_m, is a fixed value. Membrane resistance can be changed when, for example, an action potential occurs or under the influence of synaptic transmitters. We are not aware of any biological process that changes c_m in a cell. (The next chapter explains that myelin imposes a low c_m on axons, but this is a constant value for such preparations.) What does change at the membrane is the amount of stored charge (Q) or the transmembrane potential (V_m). Because C is constant, if Q is reduced by the effect of adding positive charge to the inside of a cell with an electrode, then V_m must also be reduced. This is seen as a depolarization when the inside of the cell is made more positive by our injected current.

20. Capacitative currents take time to occur and do not involve the actual passage of ion species through the membrane. Resistive currents will flow linearly and involve the actual transmembrane passage of ionic species.

21. Exponential. Yes.

22. $\tau = r_m c_m$. The units for resistance (from Ohm's law) are V/I, or volts/amp; the units for capacitance can be expressed as Q/V, or amp-secs/volt (volts/amp) $\times$ (amp-secs/volts) = seconds, that is, time.

23. A large r_m would "make it difficult" for ions to cross the membrane in response to an applied current. The ions would be shunted or diverted down the lower resistance pathway r_i, and more time would be used up getting ions across the membrane. A large c_m means a large amount of charge (Q) is held on the membrane. It will take K^+ ions more time to neutralize or discharge this extra charge before they can change the voltage and move through r_m.

24. $\sqrt{r_m/(r_i + r_o)}$. Length (or space) constant.

25. Potassium. The larger the diameter, the more internal potassium ions there will be available to carry current; this effectively means that the internal resistance is lower.

26. Neuron "A."

■ **POST-TEST**

1. No. At one length constant the local response would be 20/e = ~7 mV in amplitude. Over the second length constant it would fall to 7/e = ~2 mV, too small to depolarize the trigger zone 10 mV to threshold.

2. $\lambda = \sqrt{yR_m/(r_i + r_o)}$
   $= \sqrt{[15 \times 10^{-4}\ cm \times 5000\ \Omega\text{-}cm^2]/100\ \Omega\text{-}cm}$
   $= \sqrt{750 \times 10^{-4}\ cm^2}$
   $= 27.4 \times 10^{-2}\ cm$
   $= 2.74\ mm$

3. It is always true that when potassium ions leave the cell the membrane potential will tend to hyperpolarize or become more negative. The best example of this is the repolarization phase of the action potential. When extrinsic current is applied to depolarize a cell and drive K^+ ions outwards, as explained in the RC network analysis, the potassium leaving the cell *is* "trying" to hyperpolarize it and *would do so except that we are constantly injecting more positivity into the cell with our electrode*. The outward movement of K^+ is attempting to compensate for this perturbation. The proof of this is what happens when the current injection is shut off: as soon as the constant flow of internally injected positivity is turned off the membrane potential *hyperpolarizes* because K^+ ions *are* moving out and V_m returns to the resting level.

4. The membrane potential would not change.

5. (a) Inside.
   (b) Series.
   (c) Less at E relative to D.
   (d) Outside.
   (e) Yes.
   (f) None.
   (g) Sodium.
   (h) No.
   (i) Yes. r_m. Yes.
   (j) Parallel. Less.
   (k) No, slower.
   (l) c_m or r_m. r_m, r_i.

6. Sodium ions are now capable of moving into the cell down their electrochemical gradient because g_{Na} has been increased with membrane depolarization.

7. A receptor potential is the local response produced in the terminal membrane of a sensory axon. The size of the potential is proportional to the stimulus intensity. A simple type of receptor potential is that seen at certain skin mechanoreceptors where mechanical deformation of the terminal causes an increase in cation (mainly Na^+) permeability. If large enough, this depolarization can spread as a local potential to nearby voltage-gated Na^+ channels and initiate and aciton potential.

CHAPTER 5

Propagation of the Action Potential, Myelin, and Electrophysiology of Nerve Bundles

Concepts

1. Action potentials propagate along unmyelinated axons with loops of positive current represented by the inflow of sodium ions and the net outward movement of positive current, electrotonic on the leading edge of the action potential, repolarizing on the backside. Propagation is possible because of local (passive, electrotonic) current flow.

2. Large-diameter axons have low internal resistance, a long length constant, and fast conduction velocity of action potentials.

3. Many axons are wrapped in a myelin sheath. Myelin lowers membrane capacitance and greatly increases membrane resistance, with the net effect of greatly enhancing action potential conduction velocity.

4. Action potential currents flow only at the nodes of Ranviér in myelinated axons, and the action potential "jumps" from node to node.

5. Action potentials can be recorded extracellularly, and under these conditions they have properties different from intracellularly recorded action potentials: (a) they are small and their amplitude is proportional to axon diameter, (b) their sign is reversed, and (c) their currents sum with one another.

6. Axons are depolarized (excited) by an extracellular stimulating cathode (negative) and they are hyperpolarized (sometimes blocked) by an extracellular anode (positive). Large axons have relatively low thresholds to extracellular stimulation.

7. Normally, many axons are stimulated and recorded from together with extracellular techniques. The summed response from many axons is called a *compound action potential*. The various component responses of a compound action potential, that is, the different axons' action potentials, can be differentiated to a certain extent because of the influence of axon diameter on threshold, conduction velocity and response amplitude.

8. Action potentials can be blocked by local anesthetics, cooling, pressure, and certain toxins. With extracellular stimulating electrodes one can produce anodal block (the axons are hyperpolarized) or cathodal block (prolonged depolarization leading to accommodation or inactivation).

■ THE PROPAGATED IMPULSE

On a purely electrical basis, signals become distorted over very short distances along a cable, and one of the unique features of the action potential must be that it propagates unfailingly in an all-or-nothing manner. It must make up for the capacitive effects and the leakiness of the membrane by regenerating itself continuously as it travels along the nerve fiber. The electrotonic local currents that lead the advancing edge of an action potential serve to depolarize the membrane to threshold. The small electrotonic potentials created by the local currents are not self-regenerating and would dissipate quickly if left alone. However, by depolarizing the membrane,

they trigger the automatic mechanisms that turn on the explosive increase in sodium conductance and the ensuing spike potential. The currents flowing during the action potential then move smoothly and progressively as local currents into the next region of the membrane to depolarize it to threshold.

To examine this point in detail one can draw the action potential not in time (as is usually done), but in space, frozen in time (Figure 5-1). Knowing the conduction velocity and the duration of the action potential, one can plot voltage against distance from the center of the potential as has been done in the figure.

The peak of the action potential corresponds

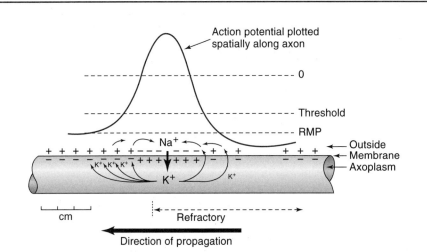

Figure 5-1 ■ Current flow associated with the propagated action potential. Depicted is a length of axon with an action potential, frozen in time, superimposed on the membrane. Above the axon is drawn the intracellularly recorded voltage change along the membrane. The influx of Na$^+$ ions beneath the overshoot of the spike provides a source of positivity to the inside of the axon that repels internal K$^+$ ions that then spread longitudinally. The local, electrotonic K$^+$ current to the left of the action potential is depolarizing regions of the axon in front of the propagating spike. The K$^+$ current to the right is leaving the membrane through voltage-gated K$^+$ channels opened by the spike depolarization. Note that the membrane is refractory to the right of the peak of the action potential, since this region of membrane contains inactivated sodium channels and open K$^+$ channels. The flow of positive current that completes the circuit includes that outside the membrane through r$_o$ that enters the region of external negativity under the spike. *RMP*, Resting membrane potential.

to a reversal of the normal membrane potential, with the outside of the membrane negatively charged with respect to the inside, i.e., during the overshoot of the spike the inside of the cell is positive. This is analogous to the situation in which positive charges were injected inside the cell with the tip of a stimulating microelectrode (see Figure 4-9). As a result, the lines of current flow will be exactly the same. Potassium ions will tend to move away from the region of the action potential. They will make the inside more positive by discharging the membrane capacitance further down the axon (to left, leading the spike in Figure 5-1), and eventually they will bring new areas of membrane to threshold and start an action potential slightly ahead of the previous one.

The K$^+$ currents moving down the axon to the right will flow out of the axon as the transmembrane current of repolarization. Note that sodium inactivation and high g_K on the trailing edge of the action potential leave the membrane (to the right) refractory, thus ensuring that the spike continues to propagate only in one direction. The key to understanding why the action potential is regenerative and non-decrementing is that the positive current, which acts as the source of the spreading local currents, is the influx of sodium that accompanies the rising phase of the action potential. This current source, whenever activated by its only trigger—depolarization to threshold—will unfailingly proceed to completion because of the built-in voltage-conductance interdependent mechanisms of the active membrane channels. If you can ever get the membrane potential to threshold, the automatic inward rush of sodium provides its own means for depolarizing surrounding regions of axon to threshold. These newly incorporated regions of membrane then become active and the sodium rushes in there, providing the source for incremental additional local currents further along the axon. Thus the action potential propagation continues unfail-

ingly throughout the extent of the processes of the neuron.

■ **QUESTIONS**   *(Answers at end of chapter)*

1. As sodium ions rush into the neuron during a spike potential, they provide a source of positive current that repels the internal _____ ions, which then move to adjacent areas of membrane as _____ currents.

2. Is it true that the electrotonic mechanisms underlying the production of local responses also serve to depolarize the membrane on the leading edge of action potentials traveling down an axon?

3. What is a major difference between the K$^+$ currents on the leading edge and the trailing end of a propagating action potential?

■ **CONDUCTION VELOCITY OF THE NERVE IMPULSE**

The action potential propagates without deterioration over the entire expanse of the cell. The rate of spread of propagation, or conduction velocity, of action potentials depends on the efficiency and rapidity at which the membrane is depolarized to threshold by local electrotonic currents. We can now immediately appreciate some of the factors that influence the conduction velocity. One of the principal factors is the length constant, λ, $(= \sqrt{r_m/[r_i + r_o]})$. As the membrane resistance increases, so the distance over which the potential falls to l/e increases, that is, more potassium current is diverted down r_i instead of passing through r_m. In other words, a part of the nerve more distant from the peak of the action potential will be brought to threshold, and the next advancing active spot will be farther away; the action potential will therefore propagate more rapidly. Two other factors that influence the length constant are: (1) the internal resistance, r_i, and (2) the resistance of the extracellular fluid, r_o. Internal resistance depends mainly on the diameter of the fiber. As the diameter increases, the internal resistance goes down. If r_i decreases, λ increases. *Thus larger axons have larger λs and conduct impulses faster*. External resistance, r_o, can influence the length constant in the same fashion as r_i. If r_o were reduced, external currents could flow more effectively and thus increase λ. However, we can generally ignore the r_o factor because the external resistance is usually very low and constant.

The time constant, τ, (= $r_m c_m$) also influences conduction velocity. In axons with smaller (briefer) time constants, local currents will spend less time discharging capacitance in any region of membrane and thus can more quickly move to more distant regions. This effect is explored in detail when the influence of myelin on action potential conduction is discussed.

Increasing the cell diameter decreases r_i and allows the flow of electrotonic currents to proceed further down the axon faster. Thus the larger the fiber, the faster its conduction velocity. Many species of invertebrates have taken advantage of this relationship and use "giant axons" in pathways mediating very rapid behavioral escape responses. Some of these axons are a few hundred microns in diameter.

■ QUESTIONS *(Answers at end of chapter)*

4. Explain in words why axons with larger length constants would be expected to conduct action potentials faster.

5. Would you expect to change the time constant by increasing r_o, i.e., the resistance of the extracellular fluid?

6. Explain how an increase in r_m, c_m, r_i, r_o, and the fiber diameter would each affect conduction velocity of an action potential in an unmyelinated axon (take the influence of each factor one at a time). Explain the relationship between fiber diameter and internal resistance.

■ IMPULSE CONDUCTION IN MYELINATED FIBERS

Except for a few rare cases, vertebrates have not used giant fibers to increase conduction velocity in their axons. Mammalian axons, for example, range from less than 1 μm to around 20 μm. However, most vertebrates have devised a special technique for increasing the conduction velocity of many of their axons, particularly the larger ones, by wrapping the axons in tight layers of glial membrane called *myelin*. Myelin is made by a remarkable process whereby certain glial cells wrap themselves around an axon repeatedly, compressing almost all the cytoplasm from between the inner surfaces of the glial plasma membrane. A tight spiral of multiple layers of compressed glial membrane forms as a cylinder closely adherent to the axonal membrane. Oligodendroglia make the myelin around axons in the central nervous system (CNS), and Schwann cells make the myelin on axons in peripheral nerves. This *myelin sheath* is not continuous over the entire length of the axon but is interrupted at regular intervals of about a millimeter along the nerve, so that the axon membrane is in direct contact with the extracellular fluid at these spaces between myelin "tubes." The small regions between the successive myelin cylinders are called the *nodes of Ranviér*, and the cylinder-sheath of myelin between nodes is called the *internode*. There is a high density of voltage-gated Na^+ channels at the *nodes of Ranviér*, and virtually none of these channels in the axon in the internodal region. It is noted that the nodes of Ranviér in myelinated axons of lower vertebrates, such as amphibians, contain both voltage-gated sodium channels and voltage-gated potassium channels (delayed rectifier K^+

channels) very similar to those seen in squid axons (see Chapter 3). Thus, at the nodes of Ranviér in these axons, the depolarizing and repolarizing currents of the action potential closely resemble those that operate in producing the action potential in unmyelinating axons, that is, the same types of channels are involved. However, in nodes of mammalian axons, there are few if any voltage-gated K^+ channels. In these axons, the repolarization of the action potential at the nodes of Ranviér relies on inactivation of Na^+ channels and the passive (electrotonic) outward flow of K^+ ions through the passive (resting, leak) channels for K^+ ions. Under normal physiological conditions, this has no significant influence on the shape or properties of the action potential. The numerous open "resting" K^+ channels are quite capable of allowing adequate amounts of outward K^+ current to occur under the driving force of the large depolarization induced by the influx of Na^+ ions during the rising phase of the spike.

The myelin acts electrically as a very good insulator—the axon membrane is effectively separated from the extracellular fluid by a lipoidal, nonconductive fused sheath of glial membrane. Thus *myelin has a very high resistance*, almost completely impeding the flow of ionic current across the axon membrane in the internodal regions. *The myelin also behaves like a large number of capacitors arranged in series and effectively imparts a very low capacitance to the internodal region*. Therefore it takes only a relatively small amount of current (potassium ions) to discharge or neutralize the capacitance of the axon under the internode.

In effect the internodal length constant has been increased and the total capacitance and time constant have been decreased, and thus longitudinal electrotonic currents will move much more rapidly down the internode.* When the axon membrane is depolarized at a node of Ranviér, the usual action potential with reversal of polarity occurs at the node (Figure 5-2). The

local electrotonic currents then flow rapidly along the internodal segment to the next node, where the full-blown action potential occurs. The internodal membrane is actually not capable of sustaining an action potential (its resistance is extremely high and there are no Na^+ channels); it simply facilitates the rapid movement of local depolarizing currents to the next node. In this way the impulse propagates rapidly down the axon, jumping from node to node; thus the name for this type of impulse conduction: *saltatory conduction* (which has nothing to do with salt but is Latin for "jumping").

The conduction velocity in myelinated fibers is much greater than that in nonmyelinated axons of comparable diameters. The relation between the conduction velocity of an impulse in a myelinated fiber and its diameter is linear. The conduction velocity (in milliseconds) can be calculated roughly by multiplying axon diameter (in microns) by six. For example, a myelinated nerve fiber with a diameter of 20 μm can conduct an impulse at 120 m/sec.

Myelination offers great economy in terms of space and the metabolic demands placed on an active nerve fiber. A nonmyelinated axon would occupy many times the volume of a myelinated axon in order to have a diameter that would permit the same conduction velocity. Because the

---

*Since myelin effectively increases r_m and decreases c_m, the question may arise how the time constant τ (= $r_m c_m$) is significantly decreased. The major reason is that c_m is reduced about an order of magnitude more than r_m is increased, so that the product of the two is still much lower than τ for an unmyelinated axon. (It is also possible to argue that since there is virtually no resistive current transversely through the internode, the only functional r_m is at the node of Ranviér. The membrane resistance there is normal, and, if this value is multiplied by the low c_m, the product yields a very low τ.) The increase in average r_m of myelinated axons is still great enough, however, to make a large increase in the length constant, λ. Also, since the largest diameter axons of mammals are myelinated, their relatively low r_i also tends to make λ larger.

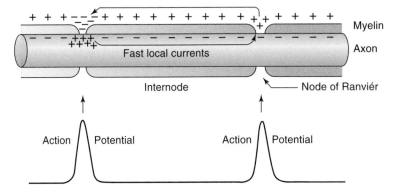

Figure 5-2 ■ Saltatory conduction of an action potential along a myelinated axon. Transmembrane action potential currents (inward Na⁺ movement, outward K⁺ movement) occur only at the nodes of Ranviér where there is a high density of voltage-gated Na⁺ channels. The high resistance (r_m) and low capacitance (c_m) of the internodal region of the axon facilitate very rapid movement of longitudinal local currents down the axon to the next node of Ranviér where the successive action potential is generated.

nodal membrane is the only area of a myelinated fiber that sustains an action potential, the amounts of sodium and potassium ions that cross the membrane will be much less than in an equivalent non-myelinated axon; the metabolic demands caused by the active transport of sodium and potassium are therefore reduced.

■ **QUESTIONS**   *(Answers at end of chapter)*

7. If you had five capacitors, all rated equally for charge storage ability, would you store more or less charge across all of them when they are wired together in series as opposed to wired in parallel?

8. All that myelin packed around an axon dramatically changes two of the electrical properties of the membrane. Which are the two properties that are altered, and how are they different from those of an unmyelinated fiber?

9. Is it true that the length constant is

decreased and the time constant increased in myelinated axons relative to unmyelinated axons of equivalent radius?

10. True or false: in myelinated axons, sodium crosses the membrane at the internodes.

11. True or false: "saltatory" refers to a pathological type of impulse propagation in patients with cerebellar lesions that make their movements jerky or jumpy.

12. When myelination appeared phylogenetically, it provided two obvious and distinct advantages. What were they?

■ **PROPERTIES OF NERVE TRUNKS**
Recording Electrical Activity in Nerve Trunks

Up to this point the discussion has been about recording from single nerve cells with an intracellular microelectrode. The potential change associated with the intracellularly recorded action potential is basically a positive-going monophasic wave. Very often in neurophysiology, we do not have the opportunity, techniques, skill, or patience to record from neurons or axons intracellularly. Therefore the electrical activity in a nerve fiber is monitored by placing electrodes, usually fine metal wires insulated except at the very tips, in the extracellular fluid very close to the nerve fiber. This method obviously does not allow us to detect transmembrane potential changes during activity; rather, it senses potential changes in the extracellular fluid resulting from longitudinal currents.

Recall (see Figure 5-1 and answer to Question 3) that the current flow associated with an action potential includes not only transmembrane currents and internal currents through r_i but also must have extracellular current flow through r_o to complete the current path for the propagated spike. With extracellular recording we are basically sampling the voltage change (E) occurring outside the axon as these ionic currents flow through r_o (i.e., $E = I \times r_o$). Although the total extracellular current is about the same as the net transmembrane current of an action potential, the former is flowing through the very low r_o, which is only a fraction of r_m. Thus the total voltage change produced extracellularly is very small compared with the transmembrane voltage change (Figure 5-3). To improve our extracellular recording (i.e., get a bigger voltage change), we can artificially increase r_o by raising the nerve into air or surrounding it with oil instead of Ringer's solution. Still, extracellular action potentials are often of magnitudes in the µV range, whereas intracellularly recorded spikes are in the mV size range. In addition to differences in size, extracellular action potentials differ from intracellularly recorded ones in that their polarity is basically reversed. In fact, because we record biological potentials as relative differences in voltage between two points (e.g., the intracellular potential is a potential relative to an "indifferent" electrode outside the cell), we can see that with

extracellular recording the baseline ("resting") potential would be zero because we are actually recording the potential difference between two electrodes outside the cell (Figures 5-3 and 5-4). However, when an action potential invades the membrane under our recording electrode, this region of the membrane becomes *negative* relative to our indifferent electrode some distance away. The negativity arises because the inrush of Na^+ ions leads to the spike overshoot and a complete reversal of the membrane potential. Thus, during an action potential, an extracellular electrode goes from zero to a small negative value and back to zero.*

Another important feature of extracellular action potentials is that, unlike intracellularly recorded spikes, extracellular ones can sum together. Axons share a common extracellular space, that is, the action potential currents all flow through the same r_o. Thus, if two or more axons have action potentials traveling down them at about the same time, the extracellular electrode will record a voltage change representing the sum of all the currents through r_o. The more axons firing, the bigger the extracellular response. Finally, one other unique feature of extracellular action potentials is that their size is also proportional to the diameter of the axon producing them. This is in marked contrast to intracellularly recorded action-potential amplitudes that are independent of axon diameter because the membrane potential is simply shifting (due to its built in voltage-dependent conductance states)

---

*It should be noted that this is a highly simplified discussion of the nature and waveform of extracellularly recorded potentials. In actuality these waveforms are more complex than indicated here; they may be triphasic in shape and are related to time derivatives of transmembrane voltage change. Furthermore, myelinated axons have even more complex waveforms, and they will differ depending on whether one is recording from a node or internode. We discuss only the fundamental features and principles of extracellular recording here.

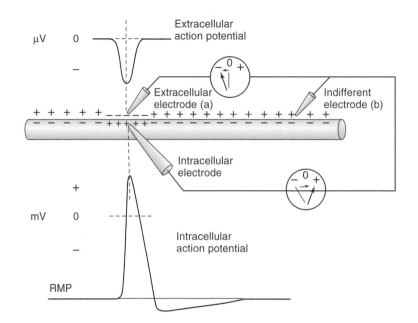

Figure 5-3 ■ Comparison of extracellular (above) and intracellular (below) action potential waveforms. An intracellularly recorded action potential is essentially a monophasic, positive-going potential change arising from a negative resting level and attaining a relatively large size (around 100 mV) that is constant. Action potentials recorded near an axon in the extracellular fluid are monophasic, negative-going waves of very small amplitude (μV range). They arise from a zero baseline, since the extracellular record is obtained from two electrodes sampling the same environment (the recording electrode (a) and the indifferent ("ground") electrode (b). The extracellular wave is negative going when the spike occurs because the external membrane is relatively negative (at [a] compared with [b]) because of the influx of Na⁺ ions during the action potential. The amplitude of the extracellular action potential is dependent on the flow of the action potential current through the low extracellular resistance r_o.

from E_K to E_{Na} and back to E_K. Because the equilibrium potentials are fixed values and the action potential simply represents a change from high g_K to high g_{Na} to high g_K, the limits of spike amplitude are fixed. However, when considering extracellularly recorded action potentials, the key variable in determining amplitude of the voltage change is total ionic current in the extracellular space. The amount of extracellular current flow is larger in larger axons, and the major reason for this is that at any instant in time more total membrane surface is occupied by a spike in a large fiber compared with a smaller one. This is seen in the following two ways:

1. Action potentials propagate down axons as a circle of activation that travels like a ring sliding down the cylindrical membrane of the axon. The larger the diameter of the axon, the larger the circumference, and thus the total area of membrane occupied by a spike is bigger and more total ionic current flows.

2. It is also known that the "wavelength" of an action potential is larger in larger axons. The wavelength basically represents the total

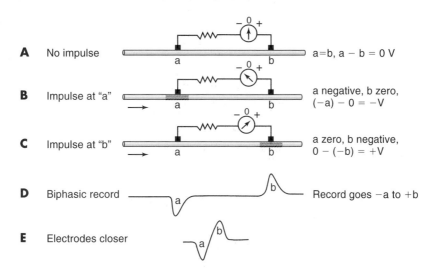

Figure 5-4 ■ Bipolar recording of extracellular action potential with two electrodes. Two electrodes some distance apart on an axon are differentially recording the invasion of an action potential along the fiber. In A the axon is silent and the potential difference between the two electrodes is 0 mV. When an action potential propagates into the area at electrode "a" (B), the recorded difference in potential between "a" and "b" is negative (D). When the impulse reaches electrode "b" (C), the sign of the recording is reversed (D). If the two electrodes are moved closer together the two separate waveforms seen in D begin to merge as a biphasic recording (E). (Modified from Brazier MAB: *The electrical activity of the nervous system*, ed 3, Philadelphia, 1968, Williams & Wilkins.)

amount of longitudinal distance a spike occupies along an axon at any instant of time (see Figure 5-1), and this value can be calculated from knowledge of the duration of the action potential and its conduction velocity. The result of this is that more total length of axon is occupied by spikes in large fibers and, again, more total membrane area is contributing to the flow of extracellular current.

The essential features of extracellularly recorded action potentials (compared with intracellularly recorded ones) can be summarized as follows: (1) they are much smaller in amplitude, (2) their polarity is reversed, (3) they can summate with one another, and (4) their amplitude is proportional to axon diameter.

The waveform of a voltage signal obtained from an extracellular recording of the nerve impulse depends on the electrode arrangement. A biphasic potential change is observed from a nerve fiber conducting an impulse if the electrodes are arranged for bipolar recording as shown in Figure 5-4, *A*. When the impulse reaches electrode "a," the region around that electrode wire becomes electronegative relative to the region of electrode "b" (Figure 5-4, *B*). (This is due, as previously discussed, to the loss of extracellular positive charge as sodium ions enter the axon.) When the impulse propagates to the position of electrode "b," this region now becomes electronegative with respect to electrode "a" (Figure 5-4, *C*). The apparent reversal of polarity is due to the fact that the electrodes are connected to opposite inputs of the recording device, such as a differential amplifier, which "subtracts" the input of electrode "b" from that of "a." Depending on the length of separation between electrodes "a" and "b," one can separate in time the two components of the biphasic wave. When the recording electrodes are separated by a few centimeters, we see two separate monophasic waves of opposite polarity (Figure 5-4, *D*). If the electrodes are close together, the two parts of the doubly recorded wave become partially superimposed (Figure 5-4, *E*).

Monophasic waves of extracellular nerve activity can be recorded by placing one electrode on the nerve and the other electrode at a cut or damaged end of the nerve. The electrodes record the potential difference between normal extracellular fluid and a more negative region where the intra-axonal fluid has been exposed due to the damage. Compared with Figure 5-4, electrode "a" would be on normal nerve; electrode "b" would be at a damaged region and sampling what is equivalent to a weak intracellular negativity. In this circumstance the baseline, or "resting" potential, extracellularly is a positive value (+a − [−b] = +a +b). When an action potential propagates under the electrode on the normal part of the nerve, this region becomes negative, approaching the negative value at electrode "b," and the potential between the recording electrodes is thus reduced. The action potential cannot invade the damaged region of nerve where the other electrode is located so that only a monophasic wave is recorded.

In our simplified discussion of extracellular waveforms here, we are treating extracellular action potentials as monophasic negative-going responses coming off of a baseline of zero potential (like the response in Figure 5-3). We shall ignore the complexities introduced by bipolar recording or by monopolar recording from cut nerve preparations.

■ **QUESTIONS**   *(Answers at end of chapter)*

13. List four ways an extracellularly recorded action potential differs significantly from an intracellularly recorded one.

14. Does the positive-going part of a biphasic extracellular spike recorded with bipolar electrodes represent that the outside of the axon becomes positive during the action potential?

15. Why is the baseline, or "resting," potential recorded by two electrodes near the outer surface of a normal quiescent axon of zero magnitude?

Compound Action Potential

It is the usual case to record extracellularly from several nerve fibers as they course together in trunks or bundles of axons. A nerve trunk, such as a peripheral nerve, will contain nerve fibers of varying diameters (Figure 5-5, *upper*). The largest axons in such bundles are excited at lower electrical stimulus strengths than are the small fibers. To see why this is so, we must consider the way in which a nerve trunk is normally stimulated. A pair of stimulating electrodes are placed onto the surface of the nerve bundle. One of the electrodes, the *cathode*, is negatively charged; the other, the *anode*, is positive. When current passes between these two electrodes, inside the cell under the negative cathode, the potassium ions will be attracted to the negative field outside the membrane. As the potassium ions move toward the cathode and up to the membrane inner surface, they will discharge the membrane capacitance, move out through the membrane, and thus produce a depolarization that can proceed to threshold. In larger axons, the amount of available potassium to move under cathodal stimulation will be greater, that is, the internal resistance, r_i, is lower in large fibers than in small ones. Thus larger fibers can be more easily brought to threshold under extracellular cathodal stimulation, and these axons will fire impulses before smaller fibers do. Therefore, when stimulating nerve trunks, a threshold stimulus is defined as one that excites only the largest

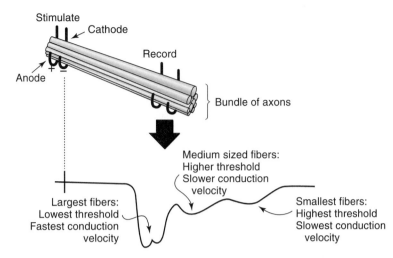

Figure 5-5 ■ Features of the compound action potential. Extracellular recordings can be made from several axons of differing diameter traveling together as a nerve bundle. Stimulation of the bundle with a pair of stimulating electrodes (an anode [+] and a cathode [–]) will produce action potentials in several axons. The stronger the stimulation, the more axons that will be excited, with the largest-diameter axons being the first to be activated. Because large axons produce the largest extracellular action potentials and conduct fastest, the recording electrodes will detect these large responses as the first to arrive (shortest latency) at the recording site. Later-arriving waves of negativity represent the contributions of smaller and smaller axons.

fibers of a nerve; smaller fibers are only activated when larger currents are given. Note that "threshold" is used in a slightly different sense when discussing extracellular stimulation. It still means adding enough stimulation strength to depolarize an axon adequately to initiate an action potential, but "threshold stimulation" of a nerve bundle means specifically the stimulus strength necessary to excite only the *largest* axon(s), not the strength required to bring all the axons or just any axon to threshold.

Recording from a nerve trunk after *suprathreshold* stimulation shows a negative wave consisting of the contributions summed together of action potentials from many active axons (Figure 5-5, *lower*). This potential change is termed the *compound action potential*. Its amplitude can be graded by varying the strength of the

stimulus. A threshold stimulation will evoke only a small negative potential change resulting from activity in a few large fibers. As the stimulus strength is increased, more fibers are excited, and their activity is added to the compound action potential. In other words, each additionally activated fiber produces a small increment in the recorded voltage created by the currents flowing in the extracellular fluid. When all the fibers are excited, the amplitude of the compound action potential is maximal; it will not increase in amplitude with further increases in the stimulus strength (supramaximal stimulation). The gradation of the compound action potential is not due to gradations in the amplitude of impulses in individual nerve fibers, since these behave in an all-or-nothing fashion.

If the nerve trunk is stimulated at a distance

from the recording electrodes, the compound action potential will exhibit several components. This is due to a time dispersion of activity in fibers of different diameters, that is, the conduction velocity is greatest in the large fibers, and impulses in these fibers will reach the recording site first. The components of the compound action potential correspond to activity in groups of fibers whose diameters fall within certain size ranges (Figure 5-5). Thus the largest (myelinated) fibers in a peripheral nerve (size range: 12–20 μm) will have the largest extracellular action potential, the fastest conduction velocity, and the lowest threshold to extracellular stimulation. Stimulus strengths of just "threshold" intensity would activate only these fibers. Additional stimulus intensity would activate an intermediate size range of fibers (also myelinated; size range: ~1–12 μm) whose extracellular spike size is smaller than that of the largest fibers and whose conduction velocity is slower. Very strong stimulation would activate the smallest axons (unmyelinated; size range: ≤1 μm), which have very small extracellular spike amplitudes and very slow conduction velocities.

■ QUESTIONS   *(Answers at end of chapter)*

16. Extracellular electrodes record a change in _____ created by the longitudinal extracellular current flow through the extracellular resistance, r_o.

17. At a point along an axon where an action potential is at its peak and sodium is rushing into the cell, the extracellular potential is (negative or positive) relative to the inside.

18. How would you manipulate two extracellular recording electrodes on an axon to obtain a biphasic wave that was continuous in shape?

19. What is a cathode? What is a cation? Why is an extracellular cathode excitatory to a nerve fiber? Would an intracellular cathode also be excitatory?

20. Explain why larger fibers can be more readily brought to threshold to produce an action potential with extracellular stimulation than can small fibers.

21. Threshold has a different meaning when it refers to extracellular stimulation of nerve trunks instead of intracellular stimulation in a single cell. How is it used in the former case?

■ CONDUCTION BLOCK

The propagation of nerve impulses can be blocked by a variety of means. Conduction block can be classified as (1) electrical, (2) pharmacological, (3) thermal, or (4) mechanical.

Electrical conduction blocks are obtained by the external application of steady depolarizing (cathodal block) or hyperpolarizing (anodal block) currents to a nerve fiber or nerve trunk. A depolarizing current may initially evoke an action potential, after which it will block impulse transmission due to local accommodation. An anodal block results from the hyperpolarization of the axon membrane, which displaces the transmembrane potential difference away from threshold. These effects are classified for extracellular cathodes and anodes; inverse but analogous effects are obtained by intracellular currents (see answer to Question 19).

A clinically useful method of producing conduction blocks is by the application of *pharmacological agents* (local anesthetics) to a nerve. These include compounds such as Novocain. Local anesthetics are thought to interfere with nerve conduction by preventing the membrane permeability changes that occur with depolarization, without affecting the resting potential. The membrane is said to be "stabilized" by local anesthetics. Small, unmyelinated nerve fibers are more sensitive to local anesthetics than are the larger myelinated fibers; they are blocked at low concentrations of the drug, which do not appreciably affect large fibers. Because of this, a differential conduction block can be obtained, which is clinically important (painful or noxious stimuli are carried by unmyelinated and small myelinated fibers). Tetrodotoxin or tetraethylammonium (TEA) also block action potentials (by interfering with Na^+ and K^+ channels, respectively; see Chapter 3), but these compounds are only used experimentally not clinically.

A transient, reversible conduction block is obtained by *lowering the temperature* of nerve fibers. This method of blocking nerve impulse transmission is accomplished by the local application of ice or an ethylchloride spray and is used clinically for producing superficial anesthesia.

Mechanical conduction blocks occur with prolonged distortion or compression of a nerve or with crushing or cutting injuries to the nerve. If the nerve membranes are not damaged, the block is reversible. Everyone has experienced a "leg going to sleep," which is a good example of a reversible mechanical conduction block in a peripheral nerve.

■ **QUESTIONS**   *(Answers at end of chapter)*

22. Describe an important clinical means of selectively and reversibly blocking conduction in small axons.

23. Cathodal block is supposed to work because of accommodation. What does this mean?

■ **POST-TEST**

1. The figure below shows the flow of positive current associated with a propagating action potential in an axon. The arrows on the loops of current indicate direction of positive flow.

   (a) The currents flowing in the region of *A* are local, or electrotonic, currents carried primarily by _____ _____ions. This current serves to _____ the membrane at the advancing edge of the action potential. The rate at which _____ ions leave the cell in this region depends on the _____ constant, which may be computed by multiplying _____ by _____.

   (b) The ions carrying most of the current at *C* or *D* are _____ ions. As these ions enter the cell in region _____, the internal membrane potential becomes more and more _____. As the membrane potential changes in this region, it is approaching the _____ equilibrium potential. A major process

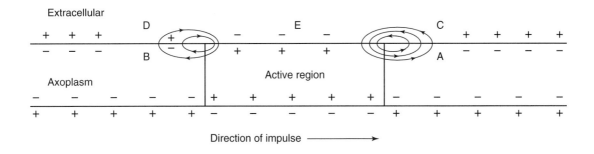

that turns off the increased conductance and inward flow of ions in this region is called _____

_____.

(c) The ions moving at region *B* are mainly _____ ions. As they cross the membrane in the _____ (inward, outward) direction, they will serve to _____ the membrane potential. The _____ of the membrane to these ions in region B is very high.

(d) If λ were increased in this fiber, would the current loops *A* to *C* be extended farther or not as far in advance of the active region?

2. If a cell wanted to reach threshold more quickly with the application of a current injection, would you increase or decrease its time constant?

3. The internal resistance of a myelinated fiber is not really different from the internal resistance of an equal-sized unmyelinated fiber, yet the former can clearly be shown to have local currents moving faster longitudinally down its axon. Why is this so?

4. Would the conduction velocity of impulses in giant axons of invertebrates travel even faster if these fibers were myelinated?

5. What is "anodal block?"

6. We have previously explained that action potentials are all-or-nothing electrical events. Explain why compound action potentials may be graded in size.

7. Experimentally, how could you spread out

the components of a compound action potential in time? Why is this possible?

8. Assume that you have two healthy normal axons; one is 1 μm in diameter, the other is 20 μm in diameter. The resting potential in each is -70 mV. (a) Which axon has the fastest conduction velocity? (b) Which is more likely myelinated? (c) Which has the largest intracellularly recorded action potential? (d) Which cell has the highest effective internal resistance? (e) Which fiber has the lowest threshold to extracellular stimulation?

■ **REFERENCES AND ADDITIONAL READINGS**

Aidley DJ: *The physiology of excitable cells*, ed 4, Cambridge, 1998, Cambridge University Press, pp 35-103.

Brazier MAB: *The electrical activity of the nervous system*, ed 3, Baltimore, 1968, Williams & Wilkins.

Chiu SY, Ritchie JM, Rogart RB, et al: A quantitative description of membrane currents in rabbit myelinated nerve, *J Physiol* (London) 292:149-166, 1979.

Hodgkin AL: *The conduction of the nervous impulse*, Springfield, Ill, 1964, Charles C Thomas.

Hodgkin AL, Rushton WAH: The electrical constants of a crustacean nerve fiber, *Proc R Soc Lond B Biol Sci* 133:444-479, 1946.

Humphrey DR, Schmidt EM: Extracellular single-unit recording methods. In Boulton AA, Baker GB, Vanderwolf CH (eds): *Neuromethods. Volume 15: Neurophysiological Techniques*, Clifton, NJ, 1990, Human Press, pp 1-64.

Huxley AF, Stämpfli R: Evidence for saltatory conduction in peripheral myelinated nerve fibres, *J Physiol* (London) 108:315-339, 1949.

Keynes RD, Ritchie JM: On the binding of labeled saxitoxin to the squid giant axon, *Proc R Soc Lond B Biol Sci* 222: 147-153, 1984.

Moore JW, Joyner RW, Brill MH, et al: Simulations of conduction in uniform myelinated fibers: relative sensitivity to changes in nodal and internodal parameters, *Biophys J* 21:147-160, 1978.

Pellegrino RG, Ritchie JM: Sodium channels in the axolemma of normal and degenerating rabbit optic nerve, *Proc R Soc Lond B Biol Sci* 222:155-160, 1984.

Ritchie JM, Rogart RB: Density of sodium channels in mammalian myelinated nerve fibers and nature of the axonal membrane under the myelin sheath, *Proc Natl Acad Sci USA* 74:211-215, 1977.

■ ANSWERS
Text Questions

1. Potassium; local or electrotonic.

2. Yes.

3. The K$^+$ currents on the leading edge of the action potential depolarize the membrane in advance of the spike by acting on the passive RC circuitry of the membrane. The K$^+$ currents on the trailing edge of an action potential are flowing out of the cell as the repolarizing currents of the spike through the voltage-sensitive K$^+$ channels (g_K is turned on by the depolarization of the spike). Note that on either side of the intense g_{Na}-dominated portion of the spike there is a net outward movement of positive current. Thus the net inward movement of positivity under the spike (mainly Na$^+$ current) is equal to the sum of the outward positive current in front of and behind (repolarization) the spike. The pattern of positive current flow associated with the action potential is thus inward in the "center" and outward in two oppositely flowing (one clockwise, the other counter-clockwise) circles on the two sides.

4. More potassium will move farther down the axon (because r_m is high and/or r_i is low) and thus will more readily depolarize greater lengths of axon in advance of the action potential.

5. No, the formula for τ, $r_m c_m$, does not contain the term r_o.

6. An increase:
   - IEn r_m would increase conduction velocity because a greater proportion of current would be diverted or used in the longitudinal direction, depolarizing more

membrane further down the axon.
   - In c_m would decrease conduction velocity because more time would be needed for local currents to depolarize the membrane to threshold.
   - In r_i would decrease conduction velocity because local currents could not move as readily in the longitudinal direction.
   - In r_o, same as r_i.
   As fiber diameter increases, the internal resistance goes down.

7. Capacitors in series store less charge (have less total capacitance) than when they are in parallel.

8. The effective membrane resistance is greatly increased, and the total membrane capacitance is reduced, compared with an unmyelinated fiber.

9. No, exactly the opposite is true.

10. False. Sodium can only cross the membrane at the nodes of Ranviér.

11. False. Saltatory refers to the segmental "jumping" of an action potential from node to node down a myelinated fiber.

12. Besides providing greater conduction velocity, myelination also affords metabolic economy, since the total amount of ionic movement across the membrane (occurring only at the nodes of Ranviér) is less and the Na, K-ATPase pump has relatively less to compensate for. Myelination provides great efficiency in terms of space, since acquiring the same conduction velocities in unmyelinated fibers would require fibers of enormous diameters.

13. Compared with intracellularly recorded

action potentials, extracellular spikes (1) are smaller in amplitude, (2) are reversed in polarity, (3) can summate with spikes from neighboring axons, and (4) have an amplitude that depends on axon diameter.

14. No, the outside of the axon becomes relatively *negative* when an action potential occurs. The waveform of the response is positive (as at electrode "b" in Figure 5-4) because our recording device *subtracts* the sign of the response under it. Since the response is negative, its sign in the recording, when subtracted, becomes positive.

15. The baseline potential is zero because both electrodes are sitting in an *isopotential* fluid; that is, the potential is the same at each electrode so that when the signal at one electrode is subtracted from the signal at the other, the result is zero difference.

16. Voltage.

17. Negative.

18. Move the recording electrodes close together (see Figure 5-4, *E*).

19. A cathode is a source of negative charges. A cation is an ion with a positive valence that would be attracted to a cathode (which is negative). An extracellular cathode attracts the intracellular potassium ions to move toward the membrane and discharge the membrane capacitance. An intracellular cathodic stimulation would be inhibitory— it would increase the intracellular negativity. (However, an intracellular anode [positive] would be excitatory; it repels intracellular K^+ ions toward the inner

surface of the membrane and causes a discharge of membrane capacitance.) Thus an intracellular anode works analogously to an extracellular cathode, and an intracellular cathode causes changes equivalent to those produced by an extracellular anode, that is, membrane hyperpolarization.

20. Because their effective internal resistance is lower, there is more potassium around to move under the influence of the stimulating cathode to discharge the membrane capacitance.

21. Threshold in this case refers to the amount of stimulating current necessary to excite the largest axons in a bundle; this is the lowest amount of stimulation needed, since large fibers are the most easily brought to threshold.

22. Local anesthetics, which selectively and reversibly block spike production in small-diameter (pain) fibers. Cooling is apparently slightly more effective for small fibers but is less selective than local anesthetics.

23. Accommodation is the phenomenon of activity block by the application of slowly increasing amounts of excitatory (depolarizing) current, which increases sodium inactivation and potassium conductance (see Chapter 4), thus preventing the production of action potentials. External cathodal stimulation applied gradually at increasing intensity for prolonged periods acts as a depolarizing current, which will cause accommodation. This is entirely comparable to passing intracellular depolarizing (anodal) current gradually and/or for long periods to produce accommodation.

■ POST-TEST

1. (a) Potassium. Depolarize. Potassium. Time. $r_m c_m$.
   (b) Sodium. E. Positive. Sodium. Sodium inactivation.
   (c) Potassium. Outward. Hyperpolarize (or repolarize). Permeability (or conductance).
   (d) Farther.

2. Decrease.

3. The myelin acts as a very good insulator, effectively increasing the total transmembrane resistance (effective r_m), thus diverting more local currents longitudinally. The myelin also acts like a large number of high-capacitance dielectrics wired *in series* with the transmembrane current path; this means that the total effective transmembrane capacitance is reduced and that less ionic current will be tied up discharging this capacitance.

4. Yes.

5. An anode on a nerve surface will block conduction because it causes an increase in the transmembrane potential (hyperpolarizes). As a positive source on the outside of a fiber, it accentuates the potential difference across the membrane and also repels or retards the movements of internal potassium ions toward the inner surface of the membrane, making it more difficult to excite the nerve.

6. Because you are recording extracellular currents flowing through a common extracellular resistance, you are recording a voltage that will vary as different axons fire and thus add to the total amount of extracellular current.

7. Spread out the distance between the stimulating and the recording electrodes because different-sized axons have varying conduction velocities, and thus the extracellular voltage changes recorded will differ as the propagated impulses cross the electrodes at varying times.

8. (a) The larger. (b) The larger. (c) The action potentials recorded intracellularly would be the same in each. (d) The smaller. (e) The larger.

CHAPTER 6

Synaptic Transmission

Concepts

1. A synapse is the site where one nerve cell, the presynaptic neuron, passes a signal to another neuron, the postsynaptic neuron. The signal between the cells is a chemical synaptic transmitter substance released from the presynaptic neurons that reacts with receptors on the postsynaptic neuron.

2. Most chemical synapses are formed by the bulbous swelling of a presynaptic axon terminal that comes into close apposition to a dendrite or the soma of a postsynaptic neuron. Synapses can also occur between axon terminals (axo-axonic) and occasionally between other parts of presynaptic and postsynaptic cells.

3. In a few cases, neurons communicate with one another through electrical synapses formed at gap junctions. Although affording rapid signaling and synchronized activity among neurons, this type of synaptic communication lacks the capability of integration and modulation seen at chemical synapses.

4. An axon can divide into many branches, thus diverging to connect synaptically with hundreds of different postsynaptic cells. Conversely, a single postsynaptic neuron can have converging upon it hundreds or thousands of synaptic inputs from other nerve cells.

5. The chemical transmitters released at presynaptic endings include a variety of small molecules such as acetylcholine, several amino acids, and several biogenic amines, and a large and diverse family of peptide transmitters. A single neuron uses only one small-molecule transmitter but may also use a peptide co-transmitter.

6. Synaptic transmitters are packaged into small vesicles in the presynaptic terminal. Vesicles are released in a statistically predictable manner when the axon terminal is invaded by an action potential. Vesicular release is critically dependent on elevated Ca^{++} ion concentration in the terminal. A complex molecular machinery is involved in the docking, fusion, and recycling of vesicles. After release from a vesicle, transmitters are removed from the synaptic cleft by uptake by specific transporter molecules that carry them back into the presynaptic terminal, by diffusion out of the cleft, or, in a few cases, by enzymatic breakdown.

7. Transmitters produce postsynaptic potentials (PSPs) in postsynaptic cells. PSPs are small, subthreshold potentials that can either excite (EPSP) or inhibit (IPSP) the postsynaptic neuron. PSPs behave like passive, electrotonic ("local") responses that spread over the surface of the cell and can summate with one another, bringing the membrane potential closer or farther from threshold. PSPs are generated by changes in ion permeability that are induced when the transmitter interacts with receptors in the postsynaptic membrane. Although short-lived, the conductance change allows specific ions to cross the membrane, moving the membrane potential toward the equilibrium potential of the permeant ion(s).

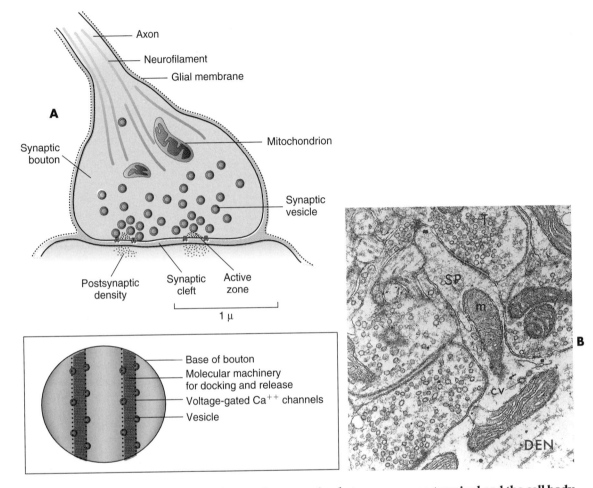

Figure 6-1 ■ **A,** Drawing of a chemical synaptic connection between an axon terminal and the cell body (soma) of another neuron. The axon terminal of the presynaptic process is bulblike or knoblike (a *bouton*, or button) and contains neurofilaments, mitochondria, and numerous spherical membrane-bound vesicles that contain the chemical transmitter. Electron densities at the presynaptic membrane, called active zones, are the sites where vesicles dock and release their contents upon appropriate stimulation. Subsynaptic densities may be seen in the postsynaptic element. These represent areas where receptors for the transmitter and associated cytoskeletal proteins may be accumulated. Synapses are typically surrounded by glial cells *(dotted lines)*, but these do not invade the widened synaptic cleft. Most synaptic boutons are only about 1 micron in diameter. The box below the synaptic terminal represents the base of a bouton looking down on it through the axoplasm. Two active zones are seen on the very bottom of the terminal, lying on the membrane as short rows. These dense areas contain molecules for docking and release of vesicles, the lateral-most part of the zone being the location of voltage-gated Ca^{++} channels. **B,** An axon terminal *(T)* makes synaptic contact with a dendritic spine *(SP).* The spine contains a mitochondrion *(m)* and its continuity with a dendrite *(DEN)* can be seen. Note the presynaptic vesicles, the wide (20 nm) and straight synaptic cleft, and the cytoplasmic thickenings subjacent to the presynaptic and postsynaptic membranes. (B from Pappas GD, Waxman SG: Synaptic fine structure—morphological correlates of chemical and electrotonic transmission. In Pappas GD, Purpura DP (eds): *Structure and function of synapses,* New York, 1972, New Raven Press, pp. 1-43.)

■ THE PRESYNAPTIC AXON AND PROPERTIES OF POSTSYNAPTIC POTENTIALS

This chapter explores synaptic transmission, the process by which neurons communicate with one another and with target tissues. In this chapter we deal mainly with the morphology of synapses, the chemical transmitters that are utilized, how the transmitters are released, and the electrophysiological properties of the potentials that these transmitters produce in the postsynaptic neuron. In the next chapter we concentrate on the receptors for transmitters, their molecular nature, and how they function to produce potential changes.

■ TYPES, ORGANIZATION, AND STRUCTURE OF SYNAPSES

The *synapse* is the location where one nerve cell makes a functional connection to another nerve cell. The typical synapse in the nervous system is composed of a *presynaptic* element, most commonly a buttonlike swelling (bouton) of an axon terminal, and a *postsynaptic* element, most commonly a small spot on the surface of a dendrite or the soma of another neuron (see Figure 1-3, *B*). The presynaptic axon terminal swelling is distinguished morphologically as containing several mitochondria, neurofilaments and other cytoskeletal elements, and a large number of small (~40 nm diameter) vesicles that contain a chemical transmitter. Synaptic vesicles are membrane-bound organelles that may be round and clear or more flattened and clear, or may be considerably larger (~100 nm) and filled with electron-dense material often representing peptides. Some of the vesicles are seen to be in close apposition to the inner surface of the terminal membrane, lying near areas of electron density called *active zones* (Figure 6-1). The presynaptic ending also contains the molecular machinery necessary to release the vesicular packets of chemical transmitter substance at the active zones

when the axon is invaded by a propagated action potential.

The space between the membranes of the pre- and postsynaptic elements is called the *synaptic cleft*. This cleft is 20 to 30 nm wide and is relatively straight; the space between adjacent neural membranes at nonsynaptic sites is somewhat narrower and more irregular in contour. Recent evidence indicates that there are transmembrane proteins in the presynaptic and postsynaptic membranes that span into the synaptic cleft and may assist with cell recognition or anchoring of the synaptic elements in proper registration with one another.

The membrane of the postsynaptic cell has inserted into it at the site just subjacent to the axon-terminal bouton molecular machinery comprising *receptors* for the transmitter substance released by the presynaptic terminal. Receptors are transmembrane proteins that have sites in their extracellular domain that recognize and bind to the transmitter molecules released from the presynaptic terminal. The cytoplasmic domains of receptor proteins interact with cytoskeletal proteins that help anchor the receptors in the proper location. At many synapses this complex of proteins can be detected with the electron microscope as dense areas just beneath the postsynaptic membrane and directly in register with the active zones of the presynaptic element. Some receptors transduce the chemical signal into a potential change (a *postsynaptic potential*) in the postsynaptic cell, but in some cases the receptors may cause other kinds of changes in the biochemical processes of the postsynaptic cell.

A common way of differentiating among synapses morphologically is to classify them by the parts of the neurons comprising the synapse. For example, if the presynaptic element is an axon, and the postsynaptic element a dendrite, or a small spinelike protrusion on a dendrite, this is termed an *axodendritic synapse*. Axodendritic and axosomatic synapses, as described above, are by far the most prevalent in the central nervous system (CNS) (Figure 6-2), but there are also axo-axonic synapses (where one axon terminal can influence the release of transmitter from another axon ending), and, less commonly, dendro-dendritic and dendro-axonic synapses also occur. Furthermore, some synapses are very complexly shaped and organized with specialized adaptations of both pre- and postsynaptic elements (Figure 6-3).

■ QUESTIONS   *(Answers at the end of the chapter)*

1. List the major morphological features of a typical chemical synapse in the brain.

2. The dense areas at the base of a presynaptic terminal that have vesicles clustered nearby are called ————————————.

The functional arrangement of these *chemical synapses* is such that an action potential propagates into the axon terminal. The depolarization caused by the action potential triggers a cascade of rapid events that cause vesicles (or "packets") of the transmitter to be released by exocytosis from the presynaptic membrane. The transmitter diffuses across the synaptic cleft and interacts with the receptors, which then induce a potential change (a *synaptic potential*) in the postsynaptic neuron. The synaptic potentials that are produced then influence the excitability of the postsynaptic cell. This kind of chemical synaptic transmission obviously has numerous steps involved and mainly serves as a transduction mechanism, via chemical intermediaries, to convert the electrical signals in one nerve cell into electrical responses in the postsynaptic neurons to which it is synaptically connected.

The surface area of presynaptic and postsynaptic cell membranes surrounding a synapse is usually covered by processes of glial cells (see Figure 6-1); in the central nervous system the glial cells are commonly astrocytes, in the periphery, at

neuromuscular junctions, they are Schwann cells.

The synapse described above is representative of the most common type of synapse in the nervous system—the chemical synaptic junction between an axon terminal and the soma-dendritic surface of another neuron. There is another type of intercellular synaptic interaction, termed an *electrical synapse*, that also exists. We briefly discuss electrical synapses here and then return to a fuller discussion of chemical synapses.

■ ELECTRICAL SYNAPSES

Electrical synapses represent a very different mechanism for cells to communicate with one another. Here, there are actual molecular bridges between presynaptic and postsynaptic elements such that electrical (ionic) current can pass directly between the cells. This arrangement is accomplished by the presence of a group of transmembrane proteins called *connexins*. Each connexin protein has four membrane-spanning domains. Six connexin molecules interact together, like staves in a barrel, to form a cylindrical complex of protein through the membrane with a pore, or channel, in the interior that is large enough for ions and small molecules to pass through. The multimeric complex of six connexin molecules forming the channel through the membrane is called a *connexon* (Figure 6-4). Hundreds of connexons are inserted side by side in a patch of membrane in both the pre- and postsynaptic cells. The presynaptic and postsynaptic membranes come very close together, separated by less than 4 nm; and the extracellular domains of the connexin subunits recognize and interact with the connexin molecules on the opposite membrane so that the connexons on both sides of the synapse are perfectly aligned and bound together. This arrangement thus creates large channels that connect the interiors of the pre- and postsynaptic cells via a continuous pathway formed through connexons aligned end to end. Such junctions between cells formed

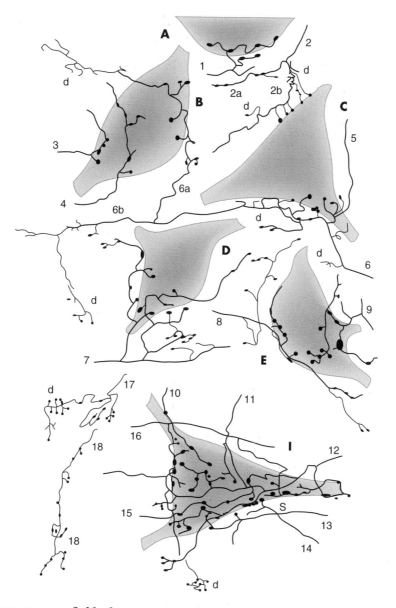

Figure 6-2 ■ Synapses on a field of motoneurons (A to E) and on a large interneuron *(I)* of spinal cord. Presynaptic axon branches *(1 to 18)* carrying synaptic knobs, or boutons, to the several cells. *d,* Synaptic knobs in contact with dendrites. Note that fiber *6* supplied both cells B and C (divergence), and that many different fibers supply each cell (convergence). (From Lorento de Nó R: *J Neurophysiol* 1:195–206, 1938.)

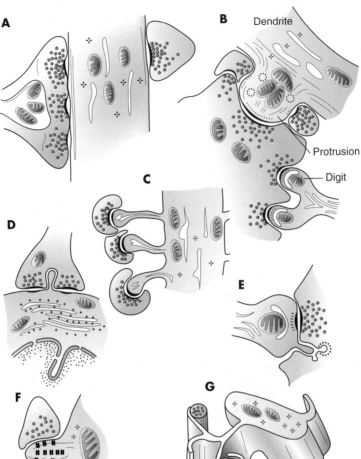

Figure 6-3 ■ Various kinds of morphologies found in certain CNS synapses. (From Szentágothai J: The morphological identification of the active synaptic region: aspects of general arrangement, of geometry and topology. In Anderson P, Jansen JKS [eds]: *Excitatory synaptic mechanisms*, Oslo, 1970, Universitetsforlaget, pp. 9–26.)

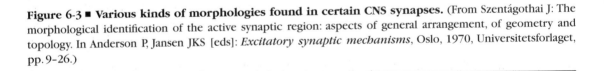

by connexon complexes are called *gap junctions.* While gap junctions are the molecular basis for electrical synapses in the nervous system, they can serve also to interconnect other kinds of cells, such as heart muscle and certain epithelial cells; cells connected in this way by

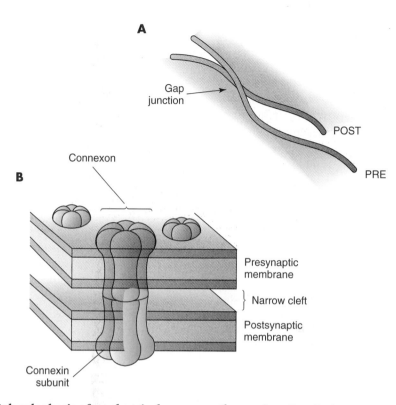

Figure 6-4 ■ Molecular basis of an electrical synapse—the gap junction. In A, two axons are shown to come into contact with one another to form an electrical synapse at a gap junction. B, Gap junctions are formed by interactions of connexon complexes in two closely adjacent membranes. Each connexon complex is formed by six connexin subunits (each of which has four membrane-spanning regions). In the center of the six connexin molecules forming the connexon complex is a relatively wide channel that is large enough to allow ions and small molecules to pass through the channel. The extracellular domains of the connexins in connexons on the opposite membranes strongly interact to hold the two connexon complexes together and thus form a bridge between the cytoplasm of the axons. Hundreds of connexons lie close together in each membrane such that many intercellular channels are present.

gap junctions are sometimes referred to as a *syncytium*. Because gap junctions allow small molecules to pass between cells, they can serve as a conduit for the passage of synchronizing signals for metabolic or developmental events. They also permit immediate transfer of ionic currents between cells, and thus electrical signals, such as action potentials or subthreshold, local currents, can pass without delay (but usually with some decrement) from one cell to another. Generally, these junctions are "two way," meaning that signals can pass in either direction. Electrical synapses are found in only a very small minority of places in the vertebrate adult nervous system but may be more common in some invertebrate nervous systems or during development. Their most obvious neurophysiological functions are to provide a means of synchronizing the electrical activity of large numbers of cells, or to provide a rapid conduction system for escape responses, where minimal synaptic delays are advantageous. Gap junctions should not be thought of as simple bidirectional, low-resistance pathways, however. Their ability to transmit current in one direction or the other is modifiable in some cases by intracellular signals, by voltage differences across the junction, or by differences in the geometry of the parts of the nerve cells that are interconnected.

Chemical synaptic junctions have functional properties that differ from electrical ones. There is no direct pathway between the cytoplasm of the two juxtaposed neurons. There is a distinct directional polarity to chemical synapses: information proceeds from the presynaptic cell to the postsynaptic one, and there is always a delay—albeit brief, a few tenths of a millisecond—between the presynaptic action potential and the start of the postsynaptic potential change because of the intervening events of exocytosis of vesicles and diffusion of transmitter across the cleft to reach the postsynaptic receptors. Most importantly, the nature of chemical synapses underlies the ability of neurons to integrate information from numerous sources and to vary their responses to multiple small, discrete input. Electrical synapses are designed to send a stereotyped signal rapidly through a series of connected cells with little integration or variability in response.

■ QUESTIONS *(Answers at the end of the chapter)*

3. A _____ is composed of many connexon molecules. Each connexon molecule has _____ connexin subunits. If ionic current moves through a gap junction, what kind of synapse connects the cells?

4. List two functional advantages served by electrical synapses.

■ SYNAPTIC TRANSMITTER SUBSTANCES

What are the ligand substances that serve as the intercellular messengers at chemical synapses? A large number and variety of chemical compounds are now believed to serve as chemical transmitter substances. All transmitters can be conveniently divided into two great families: the so-called *small-molecule transmitters* and the *peptides*. The most common and abundant small-molecule transmitters include acetylcholine, several types of biogenic amines, including norepinephrine, epinephrine, dopamine, serotonin and histamine; numerous amino acids—γ-aminobutyric acid (GABA) and glycine (inhibitory transmitters), and the so-called excitatory amino acids, glutamate and aspartate. Table 6-1 lists these transmitters, their rate-limiting synthetic enzymes, some of their prominent locations in the nervous system, and the means by which they are removed from the synaptic cleft after release. ATP and adenosine are now known also to act as transmitters at some synapses, and recently several receptors (usually designated *purinergic* receptors) for these substances have been cloned. In the past few decades a host of peptide neurotransmitters has been identified; some of these peptides (which can range in size from a few amino acids in length to those having 10 or more amino acid residues) are identical to some known peptide hormones, while other peptide transmitters are unique. Peptide transmitters include such compounds as thyrotropin-releasing hormone (TRH), vasopressin, luteinizing hormone-releasing hormone (LHRH), substance P, substance K, neuropeptide Y (NPY), several endorphin and encephalon type peptides, vasoactive intestinal protein (VIP), calcitonin gene–related peptide (CGRP), and many others.

The small-molecule transmitters are synthesized in the cytosol of the presynaptic cell. The

TABLE 6-1

Features of the major small-molecule transmitters

Transmitter	Key, Rate-Limiting Synthetic Enzyme	Prominent Location or Cell Type	Means of Removal from Cleft
Acetylcholine (ACh)	Choline-acetyltransferase	Motoneurons; autonomic system: all preganglionics, parasympathetic postganglionics, and sympathetic postganglionics to sweat glands; nucleus basalis in forebrain	Mainly by enzymatic breakdown by acetylcholinesterase into acetate and choline, the latter being taken up by nerve endings for resynthesis of ACh
Biogenic amines			Transmitter action of the amines is terminated mainly by re-uptake, although some diffusion away from the cleft also occurs. The enzymes, monoamine oxidase (MAO) and cathechol-O-methyl-transferase, while not involved in terminating synaptic actions, are important regulators of levels of the aminergic transmitters in the cytoplasm and in the extracellular space.
Dopamine (DA) (dopamine, norepinephrine, and epinephrine are all catechol-amines derived from the amino acid, tyrosine)	Tyrosine hydroxylase (via decarboxylation of L-DOPA)	Substantia nigra (pars compacta); ventral tegmental area of midbrain; hypothalamus	Uptake
Norepinephrine (NE), noradrenalin (NA)	Dopamine β-hydroxylase (from DA)	Locus ceruleus and most sympathetic postganglionics	Uptake
Epinephrine (adrenalin)	Phenylethanolamine-N-methyl transferase (PNMT) (from NE)	Adrenal medulla and brainstem	Uptake

	TABLE 6-1 *(Cont'd)*		

Features of the major small-molecule transmitters

Transmitter	Key, Rate-Limiting Synthetic Enzyme	Prominent Location or Cell Type	Means of Removal from Cleft
Serotonin (5-hydroxytryptamine or 5-HT), an indole amine	Tryptophan hydroxylase (from the amino acid tryptophan)	Midline raphe nuclei in brainstem	Uptake
Histamine	Hystidine decarboxylase	Hypothalamus	Uptake
Amino acids			
Glutamate (or aspartate)	General metabolism	Major excitatory amino acid (EAA); prevalent in many primary afferent fibers, cortical pyramidal cells and numerous other cell types and nuclei	Uptake
Glycine	General metabolism	Inhibitory transmitter; spinal cord	Uptake
γ-Aminobutyric acid (GABA)	Glutamic acid decarboxylase (from glutamate)	Major inhibitory transmitter; interneurons of cortex, striatum, olfactory bulb, retina, cerebellum (including Purkinje cells)	Uptake

enzymes for manufacturing these transmitters are in the cytosol or have immediate access to it. The enzyme dopamine β-hydroxylase, which converts dopamine to norepinephrine, is an exception to this rule. It is found only within aminergic vesicles. However, since its substrate dopamine is already provided in the vesicle by uptake of its precursor, the amino acid tyrosine, from the cytosol, this does not significantly affect the ability to resynthesize norepinephrine from cytosolic precursors. *Thus small-molecule transmitters can be synthesized anywhere in the cell.* This certainly occurs in the cell body; the newly synthesized transmitter molecules are packaged into vesicles there, and the latter are sent by fast axonal transport to the synaptic

terminal. In addition, these transmitters can also be synthesized in the terminal; and a new transmitter, or a recently uptaken transmitter, can be packaged into vesicles at the terminal. (Vesicle membrane itself is recycled in the terminal—see later section.) Peptide transmitters, which are most commonly derived by cleavage of large precursor proteins, like all proteins and peptides, must be synthesized in the cell body near the nucleus where all the synthetic machinery (RNAs, ribosomes, endoplasmic reticulum, Golgi apparatus) is located. Vesicles are filled with a protein precursor that is further processed (glycosylated and/or cleaved) within the vesicle to form one or several neuroactive peptides as it is being shipped to the terminal by fast axonal transport.

It is generally believed that peptides cannot be synthesized *de novo* in the nerve terminal, so releasable peptide transmitter must come to the terminal in vesicles via axon transport from the cell body. Each neuron has its own unique transmitter, whether it is one of the small-molecule types or one or more peptides. In some neurons there are vesicles for a small-molecule transmitter and other vesicles for peptide(s); these two kinds of vesicles may be co-released or, depending on stimulus parameters, released independently. The peptide-filled dense-core vesicles are released by a Ca^{++}-dependent mechanism that differs from that regulating release of small-molecule transmitter vesicles, and dense-core vesicle membranes are not recycled in the terminal.

To be classified as a transmitter, the compound must be *synthesized* and *stored* in the presynaptic cell and *released* from the presynaptic element on appropriate stimulation. The postsynaptic action of the transmitter must be exactly mimicked by exogenously applied transmitter chemical; and there should be some mechanism for removal of the transmitter from the synaptic cleft. For the small-molecule transmitters, the most common way they are removed from the synaptic cleft is by diffusion out of the cleft and, more importantly, by active uptake by neurons and nearby glial cells. Presynaptic endings have transporters that re-uptake a released transmitter back into the terminal for repackaging into vesicles. In the case of acetylcholine, there is an enzyme, acetylcholinesterase, in the cleft that breaks down the acetylcholine into choline and acetate. There is an active uptake of choline. Enzymatic breakdown is, however, uncommon. Even for most peptide transmitters, the evidence is not clear whether they are destroyed by enzymes, uptaken by transporters (probably unlikely), or simply diffuse out of the cleft, or some combination of these. There are enzymes that degrade amines (see Table 6-1), but these are not especially localized to the synaptic cleft. They

are widespread in tissues and the blood and serve to destroy circulating amines or amines that are in excess in the cytoplasm of neurons.

■ **QUESTIONS**   (*Answers at the end of the chapter*)

5. Which amino acid is the precursor for dopamine?

6. Where are peptide transmitters synthesized?

7. List the criteria for identifying a substance as a synaptic transmitter.

8. What is the most common manner by which transmitters are removed from the synaptic cleft?

9. How do synaptic vesicles made in the soma reach the axon terminal?

10. Name the two most common inhibitory synaptic transmitters.

■ **TRANSMITTER RELEASE**
The Neuromuscular Junction

Our basic understanding of the nature of transmitter release was first developed by Bernard Katz in England, a contemporary of Hodgkin and Huxley, who won a Nobel Prize for his work on synaptic transmission. Katz and his colleagues used as their primary preparation for studying synaptic transmission not a neural-neural connection but the innervation of frog skeletal muscle fibers by cholinergic* spinal motoneurons. Motoneurons use acetylcholine (ACh) as their transmitter, and muscle fibers express a receptor

---

*Neurons are sometimes defined with respect to the transmitter they use by applying the suffix "ergic" to the transmitter name. Thus neurons using acetylcholine are cholinergic, those using glutamate, glutamatergic, peptides, peptidergic, and so on.

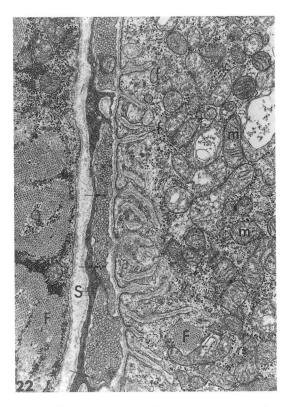

Figure 6-5 ■ **Motor endplate, or neuromuscular junction, from rat embryo. On the right is a muscle cell with infoldings *(f)*, or gutters, beneath the motor axon ending that is filled with round, clear vesicles and an occasional dense-core vesicle *(arrows)*. The terminal is ensheathed by Schwann cell processes *(S)* except at the area of synaptic contact. The intercellular gap between the motor axon terminal and the muscle fiber membrane is even wider than for an axodendritic or axosomatic synapse and is filled with the basement membrane that covers the muscle fiber. Imbedded in this basement membrane are molecules of the enzyme acetylcholinesterase, which serve to break down the transmitter acetylcholine. The muscle membrane near the tops of the gutters is very rich in acetylcholine receptors. *m*, Mitochondria; *F*, myofilaments.** (From Pappas GD, Waxman SG: Synaptic fine structure—morphological correlates of chemical and electrotonic transmission. In Pappas GD, Purpura DP (eds): *Structure and function of synapses*, 1972, New Raven Press, pp. 1–43.)

for acetylcholine, the so-called nicotinic acetylcholine receptor (nAChR), which we describe in Chapter 7. These synapses—neuromuscular junctions, or end plates (so named because the axon terminal makes a large, flat platelike synapse onto the muscle fiber surface)—are much larger than synapses between neural elements, are relatively hardy and easy to work with, and produce postsynaptic responses, called *end-plate potentials* (EPPs), that are quite large (Figures 6-5 and 6-6). In fact, the neuromuscular junction at vertebrate skeletal muscles is designed to produce a postsynaptic potential in the muscle fiber that will be large enough to bring the muscle membrane potential unfailingly to threshold and cause an action potential in the muscle fiber every time the motor axon fires. The action potential in the muscle fiber, in turn, will produce a muscle contraction. The neuromuscular junction is built to ensure that the muscle fiber contracts with each motor axon action potential, so large amounts of ACh are released to cause a superthreshold depolarization of the muscle fiber. This is in contrast to synapses among neurons, which normally produce very small postsynaptic potentials that rarely alone are large enough to reach threshold, but do permit summation and integration of multiple inputs. To study the end-plate potential, Katz and colleagues used the compound curare, purified from certain plants, that blocks the nAChR. (The toxin α-bungarotoxin from snake venom also blocks the nAChR.) This made the end-plate potential smaller and so prevented the occurrence of muscle action potentials and contractions. It was also possible to alter the ionic composition of the fluids bathing the neuromuscular preparations.

Ca^{++} is Required for Transmitter Release

A great deal of information was uncovered regarding the properties of postsynaptic potentials in these studies on the neuromuscular junction, but the two most crucial findings that have been shown to be applicable to synaptic transmission everywhere were (1) the role of calcium ions in transmitter release and (2) the quantal hypothesis. It was demonstrated that depolarization of the axon terminal is *not* the critical event that allows transmitter release. Rather, it was found that *the entry of calcium into the terminal is both necessary and sufficient for transmitter to leave the terminal*. More recent work has shown that invasion of the action potential into the terminal opens certain voltage-gated calcium channels (usually of the N-type) that are located next to the active zones. It is the in-rush of Ca^{++} ions that triggers the release of transmitter. Depolarization *per se* is not necessary or sufficient, since blocking Ca^{++} channels prevents transmitter release even when the terminal is depolarized, and elevation of intra-terminal Ca^{++} alone is sufficient to cause transmitter release, even when no depolarization occurs. The amount of Ca^{++} entering the terminal during a depolarization can be lowered by reducing the extracellular Ca^{++} concentration and/or by adding Mg^{++} ions, which block Ca^{++} channels, to the bath. The molecular details of the process of release are remarkably complex (Figure 6-7) and are under active investigation, but it is clear that calcium ions trigger reactions that lead to *docking* and *fusion* of vesicles with the axolemma (the membrane of the axon terminal facing the cleft) and *exocytosis* of the vesicular content into the synaptic cleft.

■ **QUESTIONS**   *(Answers at the end of the chapter)*

11. The synaptic response made at the neuromuscular junction is usually called an

    _____

    _____.These responses are produced by the release of which transmitter from the motor nerve terminal?

12. Where are the nicotinic acetylcholine receptors located at the neuromuscular junction?

13. What happens to molecules of acetylcholine in the synaptic cleft?

14. Invasion of the axon terminal by an action potential causes the opening of certain voltage-gated ion channels. The ion for which these channels are selective is necessary and sufficient to cause transmitter release. What is the ion?

15. What would be the effect of adding Mg^{++} ions to the neuromuscular junction?

Vesicular Release Is Highly Regulated

It has been known for some time that synaptic vesicles fuse with the axon terminal membrane near active zones, opening in an omega form to release transmitter and then "blending" into the axolemma. It is also clear that a separate process of *endocytosis* occurs near the outer margins of the presynaptic ending such that terminal membrane is budded off into the axoplasm to form new vesicles. This recycling process conserves membrane and helps to maintain a steady supply of transmitter vesicles at the terminal. New transmitter is synthesized in the terminal by cytosolic enzymes and the transmitter is pumped into the vesicles by selective transporter molecules in the vesicle membrane. The vesicles in the terminal are apparently not freely floating around in the cytoplasm. Some are held near the active zone as a readily releasable pool, immediately prepared for docking and priming for release when Ca^{++} enters the terminal. Vesicles located away from the active zones appear to be restrained, or tethered, to cytoskeletal proteins such as the actin in neurofilaments by a protein on the vesicle surface called synapsin. Phosphorylation of the synapsin by Ca^{++}/calmodulin-dependent protein kinases causes the synapsin-actin bond to be broken, and the vesicle is free to be targeted toward the active zone. Other proteins, called *Rab proteins*,

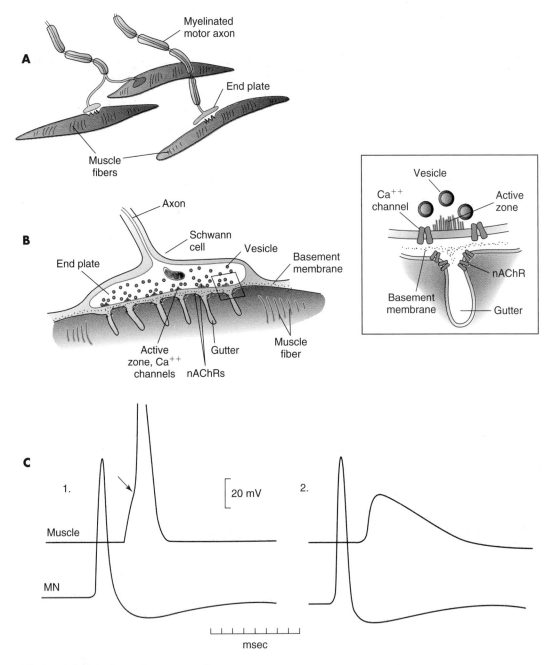

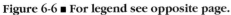

Figure 6-6 ■ For legend see opposite page.

Figure 6-6 ■ **The motor end plate and end-plate potentials. A,** Myelinated axons from motoneurons form end plates (neuromuscular junctions) on skeletal muscle fibers. **B,** Drawing of enlarged neuromuscular junction illustrating the major morphological features. The inset to the right is a further enlargement of the area boxed in the left-hand drawing. Note that the active zones of the motor terminal have vesicles (containing ACh) clustered by them and voltage-gated Ca^{++} channels adjacent to them in the terminal membrane, and that they are aligned over the gutters in the muscle membrane, near the tops of which are concentrated the nicotinic acetylcholine receptors (nAChRs). The electron density of the active zone represents the molecular machinery that, when activated by elevated intracellular Ca^{++} concentrations, will cause the vesicles to dock and fuse with the axonal membrane and empty their contents into the synaptic cleft. **C,** Recording of an end-plate potential. Shown in *1* is an intracellular recording from a motoneuron *(MN)* in which an action potential is produced. A simultaneous recording from a muscle fiber is shown above. With a short delay (latency) after the motoneuron action potential occurs there is an abrupt depolarizing response in the muscle fiber. The depolarization is caused by the opening of the acetylcholine receptors and is large enough to reach threshold *(arrow)* for a muscle-fiber action potential. The procedure is repeated in *2,* but here some curare has been added to block some of the ACh receptors so that a somewhat smaller end-plate potential is produced and the muscle membrane potential does not reach threshold. Now the pure postsynaptic event is revealed: a large, fast-rising depolarization that decays roughly exponentially after reaching a peak.

---

are attached to the outer membrane of the vesicle. It is believed that the Rab proteins, through binding of guanosine triphosphate (GTP) and its hydrolysis, may be important in this mobilization and targeting process that brings the vesicle to the proper docking site at the active zone. The docking and release process involves proteins that have been named *SNARES.* Those proteins on vesicles (v-SNARES) are the integral membrane proteins VAMP (also called synaptobrevin) and synaptotagmin (also called p65). (Synaptotagmin may not be a SNARE protein, but it contributes in a Ca^{++}-dependent manner to binding of the vesicle to the phospholipid bilayer of the axonal membrane.) The SNARES on the cytoplasmic surface of the axolemma in the active zone are called t- (for target) SNARES. One is an integral membrane protein called *syntaxin* and the other a peripheral membrane protein (i.e., less tightly bound to the axolemma) designated *SNAP-25.* When brought into close apposition (perhaps by the action of synaptotagmin), VAMP, syntaxin, and SNAP-25 form a very tightly bound complex

that likely serves to hold the vesicle adjacent to the inner surface of the axolemma, allowing it to fuse and open. The complex of v- and t-SNARES is dissociated by another pair of proteins called *NSF* (for *N*-ethylmaleimide–sensitive fusion protein, which is an ATPase) and an NSF attachment protein that is designated SNAP (but an entirely different protein than SNAP-25). With the hydrolysis of ATP, NSF and SNAP can cause the untangling of the snares. Other proteins that are likely to play a role in docking and release include another vesicle transmembrane protein called *synaptophysin,* and a protein in the axonal membrane associated with the t-SNARES called *neurexin;* elements of the cytoskeleton proper, such as spectrin proteins, also are involved. All of these proteins, along with Ca^{++} channels, contribute to the electron density of the active zone. A different set of proteins, including a protein called *clathrin* that forms a coat around a newly formed vesicle, appears to be involved in the process of endocytosis, wherein a piece of axonal membrane is pulled inward into the cytoplasm and pinches

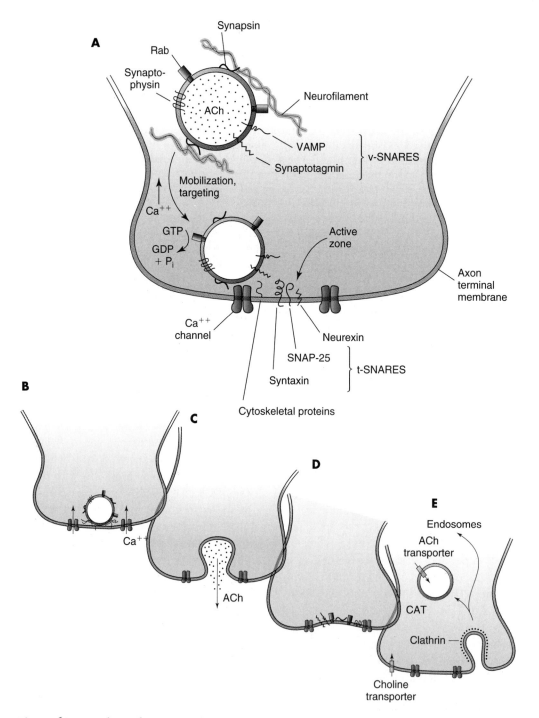

Figure 6-7 ■ For legend see opposite page.

Figure 6-7 ■ **The cycling of synaptic vesicles. A,** Terminal of an axon with an active zone containing cytoskeletal elements and t-SNARE proteins (syntaxin and SNAP-25) and bounded by voltage-gated Ca^{++} channels. In the upper part of the terminal a synaptic vesicle filled with acetylcholine (ACh) is shown anchored to the actin in neurofilaments by synapsin molecules. Also shown on the vesicle are Rab proteins and some of the transmembrane molecules believed to be involved in docking and fusion of the vesicle with the axonal membrane. These include VAMP and synaptotagmin, the v-SNARES, and synaptophysin. With elevations in Ca^{++} concentration, the synapsin binding to actin is terminated, and Rab proteins, by hydrolysis of GTP, are believed to mobilize and target the vesicle to the proper docking location in the active zone. **B,** Docking and fusion of the vesicle with the axonal membrane are triggered by the influx of Ca^{++} ions when the terminal is depolarized. The v-SNARE protein VAMP associates with the t-SNARE proteins, possibly regulated or assisted by synaptotagmin, synaptophysin, and neurexin, to bind the vesicle membrane tightly adjacent to the axon membrane. **C,** The membranes fuse, the vesicle is opened, and ACh leaves the vesicle and diffuses across the synaptic cleft to activate ACh receptors on the postsynaptic membrane. The fusion and release phenomena involve the action of other proteins (not shown), such as NSF and SNAP, to cause the SNARE proteins to disassociate. **D,** The vesicular membrane is essentially indistinguishable from axon membrane and has added to the total surface area of the terminal membrane. **E,** By separate processes, axonal membrane can be endocytosed to form new vesicles or the membrane material can be shuttled to form endosomes and be further processed. Shown in the vesicle membranes are transporter proteins that carry acetylcholine into the vesicle. New ACh is synthesized in the terminal cytosol by the enzyme choline-acetyltransferase (CAT) from acetate and choline. Choline is not synthesized in the body; it is conserved in part by being taken up by choline transporters in the axolemma from the synaptic cleft where it is produced by the breakdown of ACh by acetylcholinesterase.

---

off to form a new vesicle. The newly endocytosed vesicles can be recycled at the terminal by being refilled with transmitter, or the vesicle membrane can be fused into endosomes and eventually transported back to the cell body by retrograde axonal transport to be degraded by lysosomes.

Clostridium bacteria produce several botulinum toxins and tetanus toxin. These toxins bind to different proteins involved in vesicle release described above and block release. The toxin α-latrotoxin from the venom of the black widow spider binds to certain of the proteins to cause massive release of transmitter, eventual depletion of vesicles and block of transmission.

Quantal Hypothesis: Transmitter Is Released in Discrete Packets

Confidence that transmitter release occurs by the emptying of vesicles into the cleft, that is, that release occurs one vesicle at a time and not by movements of individual molecules of transmitter in varying numbers through the membrane, stems from the quantal hypothesis established by Katz. This theory states that transmitters are packaged in the presynaptic terminal in vesicles (a few thousands of molecules of transmitter per vesicle). These vesicles are caused to fuse with the axon membrane and "dump" their contents into the cleft whenever the adequate stimulus of calcium entry occurs. Occasionally a vesicle will fuse with the membrane and empty its contents in a random, nonstimulated fashion, causing a spontaneous "miniature" end-plate or postsynaptic potential. Customarily the action potential induces the release of large numbers of vesicles simultaneously (but independently of one another) to cause a relatively large postsynaptic event. Indeed, Katz

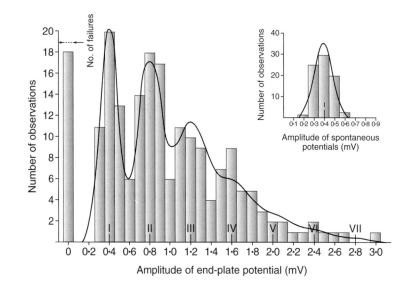

Figure 6-8 ■ **Transmitter is released in quantal packets (vesicles) in multiple numbers. The graph shows the distribution of amplitudes of end-plate potentials (EPPs) evoked by nerve stimulation at a cat neuromuscular junction in the presence of high Mg^{++}. Sometimes stimulation evoked no responses ("failures"); other stimulations produced small EPPs with sizes that clustered around peaks I-VII (smooth curve calculated from Poisson theorem) that represent the probabilities that 1, 2, 3 ... 7 quanta would be released by a single stimulation. The inset shows the mean size of spontaneously occurring miniature EPPs, believed to represent the spontaneous, random release of a single vesicle. Integral multiples of the average-sized miniature EPP (0.4 mV) appear under the peaks of the Poisson probabilities: the highest probability (I) is that one vesicle will be released, producing an EPP of average size 0.4 mV; the next highest probability (II) is that two vesicles would be released with one stimulation, producing an EPP of 0.8 mV; then a lower probability of release of three vesicles that would produce an EPP of 1.2 mV, etc.** (From Boyd IA, Martin AR: *J Physiol (London)* 132:74–91, 1956.)

and colleagues showed that with careful titration of the amount of Ca^{++} allowed to enter a terminal with each action potential, they could produce postsynaptic (end-plate) potentials that were integral multiples of the size of a single spontaneous miniature potential. Statistically, the probability of release of one or more vesicles could be predicted by Poisson theory based on the average number (*m*, the *quantal content*) of vesicles released by an impulse. Thus the smallest potential that could be induced by an action potential was the same size as a spontaneous

miniature response, and larger induced responses were found to be 2, 3, or more sizes larger than the least-sized ones: release occurred as some multiple of a single "vesicle's worth" (a quantum) of transmitter (Figure 6-8). At the neuromuscular junction in skeletal muscle, motoneurons typically release 200 to 300 packets, or vesicles (quanta), per action potential, ensuring the occurrence of a large end-plate potential that will unfailingly bring the muscle membrane potential to threshold and cause a contraction. At neural-neural synapses in the CNS, typically only a few quanta of transmitter are released per nerve impulse, causing relatively small individual postsynaptic potentials but affording the possibility of convergence of many inputs onto a cell with considerable opportunity for integration and subtle changes in membrane potential.

■ **QUESTIONS**   *(Answers at end of the chapter)*

16. Synaptotagmin cooperates with SNARE proteins to help bind vesicles to the axolemma. What are the SNARE proteins?

17. GTP is hydrolyzed by what protein to help move vesicles to their docking sites?

18. In addition to all the proteins involved in docking and fusion and cytoskeletal proteins, what other crucially important transmembrane proteins are associated with the active zone?

19. What is a quantum of transmitter?

20. Referring to Figure 6-8, in about how many times that the nerve was stimulated was only one quantum of transmitter released?

21. What is the average amplitude of the end-plate potential produced by one quantum of ACh? Would this size be altered if curare was added to the preparation? If there is an effect of curare on the size of the response, does this mean that quanta are not constant?

■ **POSTSYNAPTIC POTENTIALS**

What do transmitters do in the CNS? The best way to understand their actions is to think of them as small puffs of chemical signals that interact with specific receptors in the postsynaptic element that then cause a change in the postsynaptic cell. Commonly this change is a brief alteration in membrane permeability that causes a small potential change (a *postsynaptic potential, PSP*) in the postsynaptic neuron, but other kinds of changes can be induced as well. Most PSPs produced in nerve cells range in size from less than a millivolt to only a few millivolts in amplitude; they vary in amplitude (depending on the type of receptor, the permeability change created, and the amount of transmitter released); they can summate with one another; and they have variable durations. Based on their duration and the properties of the receptors that underlie them, PSPs are classified into two great families: *"fast" PSPs*, which persist for only a few to a few tens of milliseconds, and *"slow" PSPs*, which can last from hundreds of milliseconds to minutes to hours. Fast PSPs act on one family of receptor types, while slow PSPs act via a different family of receptor types.

PSPs are Integrated into the Membrane Potential and Alter Excitability

The function of these synaptic potentials is to alter the resting membrane potential, moving it in either the depolarizing or hyperpolarizing direction from the resting level, nearer to or farther away from threshold (Figure 6-9). Positive-going, depolarizing PSPs are said to be *excitatory postsynaptic potentials (EPSPs)*; and negative-going, hyperpolarizing PSPs are called *inhibitory postsynaptic potentials (IPSPs)*. EPSPs move the membrane potential toward threshold, while IPSPs move the potential away from threshold. Recall from the discussion of the action potential that threshold is a value of membrane potential— usually 5 to 20 mV depolarized from the resting level—at which the action potential is generated (see Chapters 3 and 5). It is the amount of membrane depolarization needed to open enough voltage-gated sodium channels to precipitate the explosive positive-feedback cycle of action potential generation. EPSPs thus make the cell more

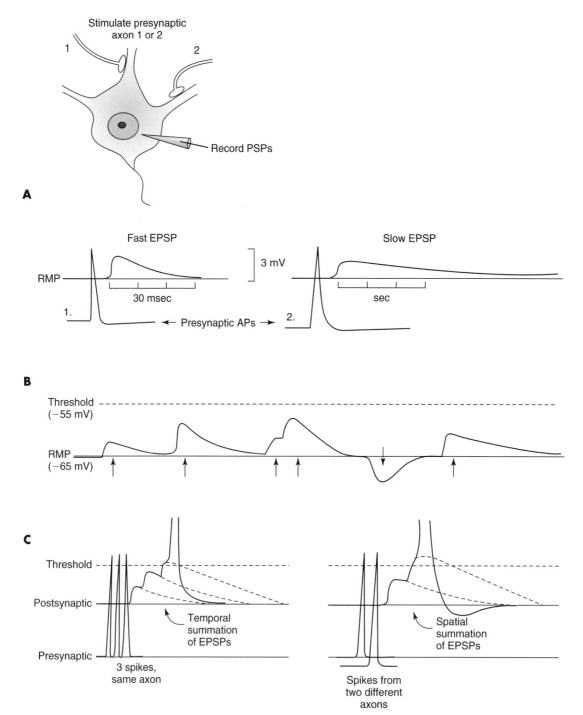

Figure 6-9 ■ For legend see opposite page.

Figure 6-9 ■ Features of excitatory postsynaptic potentials (EPSPs) and inhibitory postsynaptic potentials (IPSPs). In A, a neuron is shown receiving two different synaptic inputs (*1* and *2*) on its dendrites. As shown in the recording *(below left)*, stimulation of axon *1* produces an action potential *(AP)* that is followed with a brief latency by a "fast EPSP" in the neuron. Stimulation of axon *2* *(right)* produces a smaller and much longer-lasting "slow EPSP" in the neuron (note the slower time scale). The PSPs arise quickly from the resting membrane potential (RMP) and decay roughly exponentially. B, Intracellular recording from a neuron at rest reveals the occurrence of different PSPs produced by inputs from different presynaptic axons. The depolarizing EPSPs *(upward arrows)* move the membrane potential closer to threshold, while hyperpolarizing IPSPs *(downward arrow)* move the membrane potential away from threshold. Note also that EPSPs that occur close enough together in time can summate with one another *(middle trace)*. C, Demonstration of temporal and spatial summation of EPSPs. *Left,* The response seen in a postsynaptic neuron when the presynaptic cell is stimulated to produce a short train of three actions potential that occur at a rapid frequency. Three EPSPs sum together and actually reach threshold. The time course *(dotted lines)* is indicated that each EPSP would have had if another EPSP had not summed with it. When the same axon fires fast enough to produce summed EPSPs, this is called *temporal summation.* The summation *(right)* of two EPSPs produced by the firing of an action potential in each of two different presynaptic neurons is shown. These axons, like the ones drawn in A, generate their EPSPs at different locations on the surface of the postsynaptic cell. If the two inputs fire closely enough together in time, their respective EPSPs can summate over the surface of the postsynaptic neuron. This is called *spatial summation.*

likely to fire an action potential—they increase the excitability of the neuron. IPSPs, on the other hand, take the membrane potential in a more polarized direction, moving it away from threshold and making it less likely for the cell to fire.

Individual EPSPs and IPSPs tend to be rather small, but because of the electrotonic (RC, passive) properties of the cell membrane, these responses can sum with one another; and they do so in a more-or-less algebraic fashion. Thus, even though one EPSP may be too small to move the membrane potential to threshold, perhaps by summing with a few others it may do so (Figure 6-9, *B* and *C*). Or, just as a group of summed EPSPs are about to move the membrane potential to threshold, an IPSP occurs, taking the potential more negative and preventing the generation of an action potential. The distance over which a PSP will travel on the cell membrane after it is generated at a postsynaptic site is determined by the membrane's electronic properties, as is

the time a PSP will persist until it dissipates away. Thus, the length constant (λ) indicates how far a PSP will spread over the surface of the cell from its point of origin until it decrements to $1/e$ (~$1/3$) of its original size. Similarly, the time it takes for a PSP to decay to $1/e$ of its original size depends on the time constant (τ). Neurons that have longer length or time constants afford more opportunities for summation of PSPs and influence how readily, or "briskly," a cell responds to synaptic inputs.

Note that a single axon may divide many times into smaller branches, *diverging* to make synaptic inputs onto many cells (see Fig. 6-2). Also, a single neuron may receive inputs from many different presynaptic input sources that *converge* on that cell. Indeed, a typical neuron in the CNS may receive a few hundred or thousands of synaptic inputs. These occur at discrete locations on different parts of the cell—some ending on dendrites, others on specific places on the cell body—the placement is determined genetically and by development guidance cues. (As a rule, EPSPs tend to occur more on dendrites and IPSPs on the cell body, often near the trigger zone-axon-hillock region. It should be obvious that as a result of passive decay properties of subthreshold PSPs, the nearer the trigger zone a PSP is generated, the more powerful its influence on whether the membrane potential will reach threshold.) Thus, at any second, a neuron is processing many different synaptic inputs, integrating their effects over its surface, modulating its membrane potential, and, in effect, "waiting" to see if enough net depolarization has occurred to reach threshold, thus permitting this neuron to make its only meaningful response to PSPs: whether or not to produce its own signal (an action potential with subsequent transmitter release) for the next set of cells to which it is connected. The ability of a neuron to summate inputs from different synaptic sources at different locations on its processes is called *spatial summation* (Figure 6-9, *C*) and implies that the cell receives inputs from two or more different synaptic endings in a close enough period of time that these PSPs can summate over the space of the membrane (λ is especially important here). *Temporal summation* (Figure 6-9, *C*) refers to repeated PSPs from the same input source occurring rapidly enough in time (because of repetitive firing of a single input axon) that the PSPs can summate with one another before each dies away (τ is especially important here).

■ **QUESTIONS** *(Answer at the end of the chapter)*

22. An EPSP is seen to be 3 mV in amplitude at its site of origin. As this EPSP spreads over the membrane it will decrement in size. How large will the EPSP be after it has spread over a distance equal to the length constant (λ)?

23. Define spatial summation and temporal summation with respect to synaptic inputs to a neuron. Discuss how λ and τ

can influence synaptic interactions in the postsynaptic membrane.

Transmitters Can Change Membrane Permeability

How are postsynaptic potentials generated? The basic mechanism is that the binding of transmitter to receptor causes an opening of ion-selective channels—an increase in permeability, or conductance, for the ions. If we remember the rule that *the membrane potential always moves toward the equilibrium potential for the ion(s) to which it is most permeable,* we can see that this increase in permeability will cause a change in the membrane potential. Transmitters that bind with receptors that can increase permeability to sodium ions will consequently make the membrane potential move in the depolarizing direction—toward E_{Na} and thus toward threshold (EPSPs). These would be excitatory transmitters, as they tend to make the cell more likely to fire an action potential. If a receptor has the capability to increase the membrane's permeability to chloride or to potassium ions, the membrane potential will be driven toward E_{Cl} or E_K, respectively, values that are more negative than the resting potential. Thus the cell will be hyperpolarized, or inhibited (IPSPs). The time during which a transmitter is bound to its receptor is quite brief (a millisecond or 2 or less). Thus the period during which membrane conductance is increased is also brief. This short period sees the influx or efflux of the appropriate ionic current through the opened channel. This current (I_{ion}) passing through the membrane resistance (R_m) creates the voltage change we see as the rising phase and peak of the PSP ($I_{ion} \times R_m = V_{PSP}$). The transmitter has had little time to bind and cause channel opening when the transmitter dissociates from the receptor and the channel closes. Thus the PSP rising phase is quite brief. The decay from peak—after the induced conductance state has ceased—mainly depends on the passive RC properties of the membrane, that is, the PSP amplitude will return to baseline over a time course dependent on τ and will spread over a distance of the membrane dependent on λ. Clearly, to understand how transmitters work, we need to learn more about their receptors and how transmitter interaction with the receptor leads to a change in conductance. These are the topics of Chapter 7.

■ POST-TEST

1. Some spinal inhibitory interneurons use glycine as their transmitter. Glycine opens chloride channels. In mammals, $[Cl^-]_o \approx 125$ mM and, in neurons, $[Cl^-]_i \approx 9$ mM. At body temperature (where RT/FZ = 61), calculate the equilibrium (Nernst) potential for chloride.

2. A neuron has a resting membrane potential of –65 mV. Threshold is –55 mV (10 mV depolarized from rest). The length constant for the neuron is 10 μm. The neuron receives simultaneously three synaptic inputs: an EPSP of 10 mV amplitude produced 20 μm from the trigger zone, an EPSP of 8 mV amplitude 10 μm from the trigger zone, and an IPSP of 4 mV amplitude 5 μm away from the trigger zone. Will this combination of inputs cause the cell to fire an action potential?

3. Neuron A has a time constant of 4 msec, and neuron B has a time constant of 8 msec. All other things being equal, in which neuron would an EPSP have the better chance to add to another EPSP?

■ REFERENCES AND ADDITIONAL READINGS

Aidley DJ: *The physiology of excitable cells*, ed 4, Cambridge, 1998, Cambridge University Press.

Bennett MV: Gap junctions as electrical synapses, *J Neurocytol* 26:349–366, 1997.

Boyd IA, Martin AR: The end-plate potential in mammalian muscle, *J Physiol (London)* 132:74–91, 1956.

Cherubini E, Conti F: Generating diversity at GABAergic synapses, *Trends Neurosci* 24:155–162, 2001.

Coombs JS, Eccles JC, Fatt P: The specific ionic conductances and the ionic movements across the motoneuronal membrane that produce the inhibitory post-synaptic potential, *J Physiol (London)* 130:326–373, 1955.

Cremona O, De Camilli P: Synaptic vesicle endocytosis, *Curr Opin Neurobiol* 7:323–330, 1997.

del Castillo J, Katz B: Quantal components of the end-plate potential, *J Physiol (London)* 124:560–573, 1954.

Eccles JC: The physiology of synapses, New York, 1964, Academic Press.

Faber DS, Korn H: Unitary conductance changes at teleost Mauthner cell glycinergic synapses: a voltage-clamp and pharmacologic analysis, *J Neurophysiol* 60:1982–1999, 1988.

Fatt P, Katz B: An analysis of the end-plate potential recorded with an intra-cellular electrode, *J Physiol (London)* 115:320–370, 1951.

Fatt P, Katz B: Spontaneous subthreshold activity at motor nerve endings, *J Physiol (London)* 117:109–128, 1952.

Furshpan EJ, Potter DD: Transmission at the giant motor synapses of the crayfish, *J Physiol (London)* 145:289–325, 1959.

Geppert M, Sudhof TC: RAB3 and synaptotagmin: the yin and yang of synaptic membrane fusion, *Annu Rev Neurosci* 21:75–95, 1998.

Goodenough DA, Goliger JA, Paul DL: Connexins, connexons, and intercellular communication, *Annu Rev Biochem* 65:475–502, 1996.

Hanson PI, Heuser JE, Jahn R: Neurotransmitter release—four years of SNARE complexes, *Curr Opin Neurobiol* 7:310–315, 1997.

Heuser JE, Reese TS: Structural changes in transmitter release at the frog neuromuscular junction, *J Cell Biol* 88:564–580, 1981.

Jones EG (ed): *The structural basis of neurobiology*, New York, 1983, Elsevier.

Kandel ER, Schwartz JH, Jessell TM: *Principles of neural science*, ed 4, New York, 2000, McGraw-Hill.

Katz B: *The release of neural transmitter substance*, Springfield, Ill, 1969, Charles C Thomas.

Katz B, Miledi R: The study of synaptic transmission in the absence of nerve impulses, *J Physiol (London)* 192:407–436, 1967.

Katz B, Miledi R: The timing of calcium action during neuromuscular transmission, *J Physiol (London)* 189:535–544, 1967.

Liley AW: The quantal components of the mammalian end-plate potential, *J Physiol (London)* 133:571–587, 1956.

Llinas RR: Calcium in synaptic transmission, *Sci Am* 247: 56-65, 1982.

Llinas RR, Steinberg IZ, Walton K: Relationship between presynaptic calcium current and postsynaptic potential in squid giant synapse, *Biophys J* 33:323-351, 1981.

Lorento de Nó R: Synaptic stimulation of motoneurons as a local process, *J Neurophysiol* 1:195-206, 1938.

Neher E, Sakmann B: Single-channel currents recorded from membrane of denervated frog muscle fibers, *Nature* 260:799-802, 1976.

Nicholls JG, Martin AR, Wallace BG, et al: *From neuron to brain*, ed 4, Sunderland, Mass, 2001, Sinauer Associates.

Pappas GD, Waxman SG: Synaptic fine structure—morphological correlates of chemical and electrotonic transmission. In Pappas GD, Purpura DP (eds): *Structure and function of synapses*, 1972, New Raven Press, pp. 1-43.

Peters A, Palay SL, Webster H deF: *The fine structure of the nervous system: the neurons and supporting cells*, Philadelphia, 1976, WB Saunders.

Redman S: Quantal analysis of synaptic potentials in neurons of the central nervous system, *Physiol Rev* 70:165-198, 1990.

Robitaille R, Adler EM, Charlton MP: Strategic location of calcium channels at transmitter release sites of frog neuromuscular synapses, *Neuron* 5:773-779, 1990.

Scheller RH: Membrane trafficking in the presynaptic nerve terminal, *Neuron* 14:893-897, 1995.

Schweizer FE, Betz H, Augustine GJ: From vesicle docking to endocytosis: intermediate reactions of exocytosis, *Neuron* 14:689-696, 1995.

Smith SJ, Augustine GJ: Calcium ions, active zones and synaptic transmitter release, *Trends Neurosci* 11:458-464, 1988.

Söllner T, Whiteheart SW, Brunner M, et al: SNAP receptors implicated in vesicle targeting and fusion, *Nature* 362: 318-324, 1993.

Sudhof TC : The synaptic vesicle cycle: a cascade of protein-protein interactions, *Nature* 375:645-653, 1995.

Sudhof TC, Czernik AJ, Kao H-T, et al: Synapsins: mosaics of shared and individual domains in a family of synaptic vesicle phosphoproteins, *Science* 245:1474-1480, 1989.

Szentágothai J: The morphological identification of the active synaptic region: aspects of general arrangement, of geometry and topology. In Anderson P, Jansen JKS (eds): *Excitatory synaptic mechanisms*, Oslo, 1970, Universitetsforlaget, pp. 9-26.

Takeuchi A, Takeuchi N: On the permeability of the end-plate membrane during the action of transmitter, *J Physiol (London)* 154:52-67, 1960.

von Gersdorff H, Matthews G: Dynamics of synaptic vesicle fusion and membrane retrieval in synaptic terminals, *Nature* 367:735-739, 1994.

Zigmond MJ, Bloom FE, Roberts JL, et al (eds): *Fundamental neuroscience*, New York, 1999, Academic Press.

■ ANSWERS
Text Questions

1. The typical chemical synapse is composed of a bulblike axon terminal and the dendrite of another neuron. The presynaptic terminal is characterized by neurofilaments, mitochondria and, especially, vesicles. The synaptic cleft is relatively wide and straight. Receptors are located postsynaptically near areas of postsynaptic densities.

2. Active zones.

3. Gap junctions. Six.

4. Synchronizing electrical activity; allowing rapid transmission of signals among neurons.

5. Tyrosine.

6. In the cell body; they cannot be synthesized in the terminal.

7. Must be synthesized and stored in the presynaptic terminal; must be released with appropriate stimulation; must be mimicked in its actions by exogenously applied transmitter; must have a specific mechanism for removing it from the synaptic cleft.

8. Re-uptake into axon terminals. Transmitters can also be taken up by glial cells and by postsynaptic cells.

9. Synaptic vesicles, like many other cellular organelles (e.g., mitochondria) reach the axon terminal by fast axonal transport.

10. GABA and glycine.

11. End-plate potential (EPP). Acetylcholine.

12. In the membrane of the muscle fiber at the tops of the folds, or gutters, just beneath the active zones of the motor nerve terminal.

13. Some diffuse out of the cleft. Others react with the acetylcholine receptors but then dissociate from the receptors. Most of the ACh molecules are broken down into choline and acetate in the cleft by the enzyme acetylcholinesterase, which is imbedded in the basement membrane in the cleft of the junction. The choline is actively taken up by transporter molecules in the membrane of the motor terminal.

14. Ca^{++}.

15. Addition of Mg^{++} ions would prevent Ca^{++} entry into the nerve terminal and thus reduce the number of vesicles of transmitter that could be released. The end-plate potential would be smaller under these conditions.

16. The v-SNARE protein on the vesicle is called VAMP (or synaptobrevin); the t-SNARES on the axolemmal membrane are called syntaxin and SNAP-25. VAMP and syntaxin are integral membrane proteins; SNAP-25 a peripheral membrane protein.

17. The RAB proteins hydrolyze GTP and so assist in moving the vesicle to the docking site.

18. Voltage-gated Ca^{++} channels. Commonly these are the N-type, but in some cases P/Q calcium channels may be present.

19. A quantum of transmitter is the amount of transmitter in one vesicle.

20. The Poisson equation predicted that in this experiment there should have been about 20 times that a stimulation would release one quantum (or vesicle) of transmitter. This is shown by the peak of the smooth theoretical Poisson curve at the ordinate value of 20 and the potential size of 0.4 mV, also labeled "I" on the graph. In 11 stimulations a potential of amplitude 0.3 mV was evoked, and on 13 stimulations potentials of 0.5 mV were evoked. These probably also represent trials when only one vesicle was released, but the amplitude varied a bit because of electrical noise.

21. The average amplitude of the EPP produced by one quantum (or vesicle) of transmitter is 0.4 mV. This was seen in two ways: first, this was the mean amplitude of spontaneously released miniature EPPs; and, second, it was the mean size of the smallest EPP produced by nerve stimulation. If curare were added to the preparation, the size of the EPPS, whether spontaneous or induced, would be smaller. This does not mean that the amount of transmitter released was reduced, that is, that the size of a quantum got smaller; it simply means that fewer ACh receptors were available to interact with the transmitter, so a smaller response occurred.

22. The initial EPSP (V_o = 3 mV) will decrement to approximately 1 mV after it travels a distance equal to the length constant λ. The amplitude of the EPSP after it has traveled distance x will be V_x. $V_x = V_o e^{-x/\lambda}$. When the distance x = λ, then $V_x = V_o e^{-1} = V_o/e = 3mV/e = \sim 1$ mV.

23. **Spatial summation:** inputs from two or more *different* presynaptic endings are close enough together on the membrane surface of the postsynaptic cell to be able to

summate with one another over the space of the membrane before either dissipates to zero. **Temporal summation:** repetitive inputs from the *same* presynaptic ending occur fast enough to be able to summate in time before either dissipates to zero.

The length (or space) constant (λ): determines how *far* a PSP will travel before it dissipates to l/e of its original size. The larger λ is, the more opportunities a PSP will have to summate with another PSP generated at a different ending on the membrane surface.

The time constant (τ): determines how *long* (*for what duration*) any PSP will persist on the membrane before it dissipates to l/e of its original size. The larger τ is, the more opportunities a PSP caused by a single ending will have to add to another PSP produced at the same ending (or to PSPs produced elsewhere on the postsynaptic surface).

■ POST-TEST

1. $E_{Cl} = RT/FZ \ln \{[Cl^-]_i/[Cl^-]_o\}$
   $= 61 \log_{10} \{9/125\}$
   $= 61 \log_{10} (0.072)$
   $= 61 (-1.143)$
   $= -69.7$ mV

2. The answer is no. The calculations are as follows. We will need to determine the size of each of the PSPs after it has traveled its respective distance from site of initiation to the trigger zone ($V_x = V_o e^{-x/\lambda}$). The 8 mV EPSP must travel a distance equal to the length constant of the cell (10 μm). For it, $V_x = 8\ e^{-10/10} = 8\ e^{-1} = 8(0.367) = 2.9$ mV, the size of the EPSP when it arrives at the trigger zone. For the 10 mV EPSP that is 20 μm away from the trigger zone, $V_x = 10e^{-20/10} = 10e^{-2} = 10\ (0.135) = 1.35$ mV, its size when it reaches the trigger zone. For the IPSP, $V_x = 5e^{-5/10} = 5e^{-0.5} = 5(0.61) = 2.44$ mV. Since this last PSP is inhibitory, its sign is negative (it is a hyperpolarizing response), so the IPSP will be -2.44 mV at the trigger zone. At the trigger zone the three PSPs will add algebraically, so the change in membrane potential will be 2.9 mV + 1.35 mV -2.44 mV, or a net change in membrane potential of 1.8 mV. This means the cell would be depolarized by 1.8 mV from rest. This is less than the 10 mV needed to reach threshold, so no action potential will occur.

3. Neuron B. EPSPs that occur in a cell with a longer time constant will last longer before they decrement away, so there would be more opportunity to sum with another PSP.

CHAPTER 7

Synaptic Transmission: Receptors and Their Actions

Concepts

1. The postsynaptic receptors for chemical transmitters belong to two great families based on their molecular structure and functional properties.

2. One family of receptors is called *directly gated ionotropic receptors* and accounts for a class of synaptic responses called *fast postsynaptic potentials (PSPs)*. These receptors have a molecular structure comprising 3 to 5 protein subunits that span the membrane. Certain subunits contain binding sites for the transmitter on their extracellular surface, and all the subunits form a channel, or ionophore, through the membrane that is selective for specific ions. Binding of transmitter induces conformational changes in the subunits that open the ionophore and allow the appropriate ions to move in or out of the cell along their electrochemical gradients.

3. The increase in permeability (conductance) to ions at ionotropic receptors is thus directly gated by the ligand transmitter. The ionophore is open for only a brief time, producing a fast PSP. If the ionophore is selective for Na^+ ions, they would move into the cell, causing a depolarization and bringing the cell nearer to threshold. Such responses are called *excitatory postsynaptic potentials (EPSPs)*. The gated opening of ionophores selective for Cl^- or K^+ ions would cause negative-going changes in membrane potential, taking the cell away from threshold or making the cell less excitable; such responses are *inhibitory postsynaptic potentials (IPSPs)*.

Because the membrane potential always moves toward the equilibrium potential for the ion(s) to which the cell is most permeable, one can always predict the change in membrane potential during transmitter action if we know which ion's permeability is being increased by the transmitter action.

4. The so-called nicotinic acetylcholine receptor (nAChR) at the neuromuscular junction is the prototypic ionotropic receptor. This preparation has served as a model for understanding the process of transmitter release and the structure and properties of "fast" receptors and fast PSPs. The features of fast synaptic transmission at neural-neural synapses are comparable to transmission at the neuromuscular junction, but unlike the very large postsynaptic response (often called an *end-plate potential [EPP]*) produced at the neuromuscular junction, the PSPs produced in neurons are very small. Neuronal PSPs can summate with one another because of the RC circuitry of the passive membrane. Converging inputs produce PSPs that are continuously being integrated into the membrane potential, moving the resting potential nearer or farther from threshold and regulating the action potential output of the postsynaptic cell.

5. A second great class of postsynaptic receptors is entirely different from the directly-gated, multimeric ionotropic ones that account for fast PSPs. They are designated metabotropic receptors and belong to a class of

135

genetically related proteins: each is a large continuous protein that has seven membrane-spanning domains. They do not form channels. Rather, they are associated with G-proteins (named for their affinity for guanosine nucleotides) in the inner leaflet of the postsynaptic membrane. Binding of transmitter induces conformational changes in the receptor, which then associates with G-protein subunits. This initiates a cascade of biochemical events: a G-protein subunit now binds GTP and activates effector proteins (usually enzymes) that produce second messenger molecules that have diverse, widespread, and persistent actions on many different aspects of postsynaptic metabolism or postsynaptic potential production.

6. One set of possible outcomes of activation of certain of these receptors is the production of slow PSPs. The second messenger cascades can influence the opening or closing of channels in the membrane that permit ionic synaptic currents. These channel effects have a slow time course and are relatively long lasting, persisting for seconds to many hours.

7. Activation of other metabotropic receptors can also cause, via other cascades, changes in the properties of voltage-gated ion channels, thus altering the shape and duration of action potentials. These receptors can also induce a host of biochemical and metabolic alterations in neurons, including gene transcription and resultant long-term changes in cell function and structure.

■ IONOTROPIC RECEPTORS

Ionotropic Receptors Are Multimeric Receptor-Channel Complexes

The family of receptors associated with "fast" PSPs has a coherent set of properties that account for their selective binding with specific ligands (transmitters), rapid action, and their selectivity for ion permeation. All of these receptors are called *ionotropic* receptors because their molecular structure incorporates both the "receptor" part of the molecular complex and an ion channel, or *ionophore*. The most thoroughly studied ionotropic receptor is the nicotinic acetylcholine receptor (nAChR) at the neuromuscular junction discussed in Chapter 6 (the accessibility and abundance of this receptor have made its isolation and purification easiest). However, all ionotropic receptors are structurally and genetically related. The nAChR is also found on some neurons in the autonomic and central nervous systems. A model of the muscle receptor is shown in Figure 7-1 as a prototype for most of the ionotropic receptor-channel complexes that underlie fast EPSPs. The nAChR receptor-ionophore complex contains five subunits: two alphas (α) and one each of beta (β), gamma (γ), and delta

(δ). (In developing nervous systems, the δ subunit is substituted by a different subunit called epsilon (ϵ); on different neurons and skeletal muscles various isoforms of the subunits are commonly found.) Each of the subunits has multiple transmembrane α-helices; the four membrane spanning domains (M1 to M4) of the α subunit are shown in Figure 7-1, *A;* the transmembrane domains of the other subunits have considerable homology to those of the α subunit. Part of the amino acid sequence of the extracellular domain of each of the α subunits is the specific binding site for acetylcholine (ACh); one molecule of ACh must bind to each α subunit to activate (open) the channel. All of the subunits interact to form a relatively large (compared with voltage-gated channels for Na$^+$ or K$^+$ ions) hydrophilic channel through the lipoidal membrane, which is said to be *cation-selective,* that is, the channel is permeable to Na$^+$ *and* K$^+$ ions and can even allow some Ca^{++} through (Figure 7-1, *B*). When ACh binds to the α subunits, the ensemble of subunits changes its conformation, opening the channel. The M2 domains of the five subunits lie nearest the center of the channel, forming its walls, and are probably critical for transducing the opening

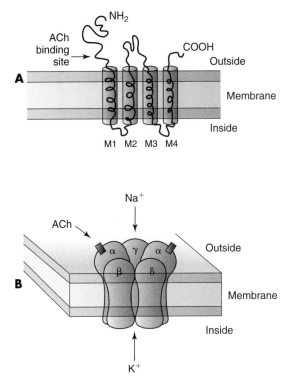

Figure 7-1 ■ **The nicotinic acetylcholine receptor (nAChR). A,** Drawing of the α subunit of the receptor with its topology in the membrane. Four transmembrane domains (M1–M4) are formed by α-helices. The *N*-terminal of the protein in the extracellular space contains the acetylcholine binding site. The other subunits of the ACh receptor share considerable homology to the α subunit. **B,** Rendition of the entire nAChR in the membrane with the five subunits (two α subunits and one each of β, γ, and δ) organized to form a cationic channel in the center. The M2 domain of each subunit is aligned to line the channel. An ACh binding site is depicted on each α subunit. Binding of ACh opens the channel, which is equally permeable to Na$^+$ and K$^+$ ions. These ions move through the channel under the influence of their respective electrochemical gradients.

conformational change induced by ACh. Sodium and potassium ions then move through the channel in strict accordance to the electrochemical driving forces on each ion.

Ionotropic Ionophores Have Ion Selectivity

At the normal resting potential of a nerve or muscle cell (–60 to –90 mV), the inwardly directed electrochemical driving force on Na$^+$ ions is strong. The amount of inward Na$^+$ current, I_{Na}, would be equal to the sodium conductance, g_{Na}, times the electrical driving force ($V_m - E_{Na}$). With a resting potential of –70 mV (V_m) and a value of +55 mV for E_{Na}, the electrical force pulling sodium ions into the cell is some –125 mV; so, for a particular conductance increase, there should be a large inward sodium current that would make the inside of the cell more positive. An equal increase in conductance for K$^+$ ions, g_K, would produce a relatively very small outward K$^+$ current, since the electrical driving force to repel K$^+$ ions from the interior of the cell is small: ($V_m - E_K$) = –70 – (–75) = +5 mV. This small outward potassium current would tend to make the inside of the cell slightly more negative, an opposite effect of the inward sodium movement. Thus, at the outset of the transmitter action, the *net* effect on the cell would be a large influx of positive current that would *depolarize* V_m. If acetylcholine does open a channel that is equally permeable to Na$^+$ and K$^+$ ions, we can predict just how large the depolarization would be if we left the transmitter on for a long time, permitting the membrane potential to move to a steady-state value based on the cell having equal conductances to Na$^+$ and K$^+$ ions. When $g_{Na} = g_K$, the membrane potential, in attempting to move to the equilibrium potential for the ions to which it is most permeable, will move to a value that is halfway between E_{Na} and E_K:

$$(E_{Na} + E_K)/2 = (+55 + [-75])/2 = -20/2 = -10 \text{ mV}$$

In a normal muscle fiber one cannot deter-

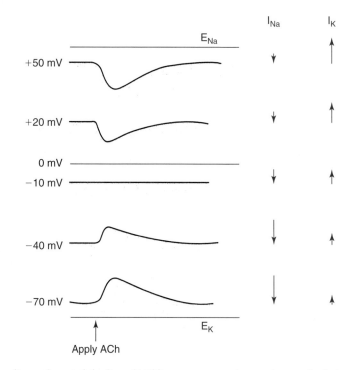

Figure 7-2 ■ **Recording of acetylcholine (ACh) responses at a motor end plate to demonstrate the reversal potential for the transmitter.** Recordings are made from a skeletal muscle fiber with a technique called *current clamp*, wherein constant-current pulses can be passed through the fiber membrane to change its potential to different values for a short time. A constant amount of ACh is applied to the same place on the fiber at the different membrane potentials. Shown in the left column are the responses to ACh at potentials starting near the resting level (–70 mV) and at increasing levels of depolarization. The ACh-induced responses become smaller as we depolarize (–40 mV). No change in membrane potential is seen when ACh is applied at the –10 mV membrane potential. At more depolarized potentials, the ACh response is inverted, going more negative as we depolarize further. The nAChR ionophore opened by ACh is equally permeable to Na$^+$ and K$^+$ ions, but the fluxes of these ions are in opposite directions and of different magnitudes, depending on the electrochemical driving force on each at each of the different membrane potentials. The columns to the right of the end-plate recordings illustrate the direction and magnitude of Na$^+$ and K$^+$ currents at each level of recorded membrane potential. Note that at –10 mV, the *reversal potential*, the Na$^+$ and K$^+$ ion movements are equal and opposite—there is no net current across the membrane, so a potential change cannot be induced by ACh at this level of membrane potential. (The 0 mV potential level is shown only for reference; no ACh was applied at this membrane potential. Had it been, the response would have been a small negative-going potential change.)

mine whether the application of ACh actually makes the membrane potential move to –10 mV because the large depolarization reaches threshold and an action potential is generated, obscuring the peak of the EPP. The problem can be approached by using a procedure referred to as *current clamp* (Figure 7-2). The membrane potential can be changed to any value by injecting a constant positive or negative current into the cell. To avoid action potentials and muscle contractions, tetrodotoxin can be added to the bath to block voltage-gated Na^+ channels. If a small of amount of ACh is squirted on when the membrane potential is held near rest at –70 mV, a small EPP is produced. Note that the currents that produce the EPP are illustrated to represent a large inward sodium current and a small outward potassium current. If enough positive clamp current is added to passively take the membrane potential to –40 mV and the same amount of ACh is applied, the EPP is smaller. The inward Na^+ current is smaller and the outward K^+ current is larger because we have moved 30 mV closer to E_{Na} (reducing the inward electrical driving force on Na^+ ions) and 30 mV farther from E_K (increasing the outward driving force on K^+ ions by reducing the electrical gradient holding them inside). At –10 mV, even though ACh is applied as before, there is no potential change in the muscle fiber. There is, of course, still the same conductance increase, but there is no *net* movement of current across the membrane: the inward Na^+ current is exactly balanced by an equal amount of outward K^+ current. At more positive values of membrane potential, the voltage change induced by ACh is *reversed*. The EPP is actually negative going. Clearly, this occurs because the outward K^+ current exceeds the inward Na^+ current, the more so as we approach E_{Na} and move farther from E_K. The membrane potential at which a transmitter does not produce a voltage change, where inward and outward currents are equal, or where the induced potential

reverses sign (all equivalent statements) is called the *reversal potential* for that transmitter. The reversal potential for acetylcholine, ACh_r, is thus approximately –10 mV in skeletal muscle fibers. In general, all cationic channels have roughly the same reversal potential because most are about equally permeable to Na^+ and K^+.

The nAChR has also been examined using the patch clamp method (Figure 7-3). It is possible to record from a single or a few nAChRs from muscle fibers with patch pipettes, and to record the current movements through a single channel when small amounts of ACh are introduced to the pipette. The patch of membrane can be voltage clamped to various potentials and the effect on ACh-induced transmembrane current through the channel observed. Plotting the amplitude of single pulses of channel current obtained at different membrane potentials produces a current-voltage (I-V) relationship that reveals both the reversal potential and the single-channel conductance (about 30 pS) for the nAChR ionophore. The conductance of these channels is larger than that for voltage-gated Na^+ or K^+ channels, reflecting the larger size of the channel and its ability to pass Na^+ and K^+ ions.

Knowing the reversal potential for a transmitter is a clue as to the ions whose conductance has been turned on by that transmitter. As with recordings of EPPs from intact muscle fibers, it can be shown that alterations in either Na^+ or K^+ ion concentrations in the extracellular fluid, which produce changes in E_{Na} and E_K, produce predictable changes in the reversal potential for single-channel currents. If $[Na^+]_o$ is reduced by half, a sodium equilibrium potential of about +38 mV (instead of the normal +55 mV) is generated. The average of this value and E_K (–75 mV) is approximately –18 mV, the new reversal potential for ACh under this condition of lowered extracellular Na^+ concentration. A plot of the currents recorded in half-normal outside Na^+ concentration is shown as the dotted

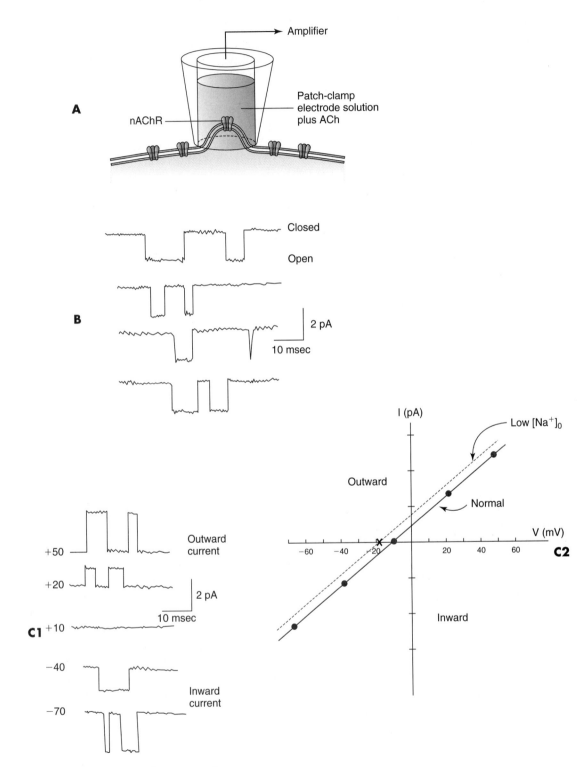

Figure 7-3 ■ For legend see opposite page.

Figure 7-3 ■ Patch-clamp recording of currents through single ionotropic nicotinic acetylcholine receptors (nAChR). A, A patch pipette is attached to a patch of membrane containing an nAChR receptor. The patch of membrane containing the receptor can be voltage-clamped to any desired potential, and ACh can be added to the electrode solution in small concentrations (around 1 μm). B, Drawing of current records obtained from the patch when ACh is present. Note that there are discrete openings of the nAChR ionophore that allow pulses of current to flow that are of constant size but of variable durations. Each downward deflection represents a pulse of net inward current through the channel. C, *1*, The membrane patch is voltage-clamped to different potentials, and ACh is added to the pipette. Brief openings of the channel are seen, but the magnitude and direction of current flow through the channel change with depolarizing clamp levels. Note that there is no net current through the membrane at –10 mV. This is the reversal potential as described in Figure 7-2 and is a direct demonstration of the lack of net current movement at this unique value. We can plot in a current-voltage (I-V) relationship (C, *2*) the magnitude and direction of current through the channel as recorded at different membrane potentials. The dots represent the values obtained in the experiment in C, *1*. The solid line through these points has a slope that represents the conductance of a single nAChR ($g_{ACh} = I_{ACh} / V$). The dotted line parallel and to the left of the solid line represents the I-V relationship that would be obtained if the experiment were repeated with an extracellular Na^+ ion concentration half the normal value (see text). The "×" on the dotted line is at ~–18 mV, the ACh_r calculated for this value of $[Na^+]_o$.

---

line in Figure 7-3, *C, 2*. The recorded reversal potential is at ~–18 mV, and the I-V relationship is parallel to the normal one but shifted leftward, a result expected if the channel is equally conductive to Na^+ and K^+ ions. Additional examples are shown later of reversal potentials for transmitters that open channels exclusively permeable to Cl^- and K^+.

■ **QUESTIONS**   *(Answers at the end of the chapter)*

1. What is an ionophore?

2. How many separate subunits are there in the nAChR? Which subunits bind ACh? Which contribute to the formation of the ionophore?

3. Define "reversal potential."

4. If the nAChR at the neuromuscular junction opens ionophore channels equally permeable to sodium and potassium ions, the reversal potential for

ACh (ACh_r) can be determined by application of the Goldman equation. Use the following values for a mammalian preparation to calculate ACh_r: $[Na^+]_o = 150$ mM; $[Na^+]_i = 15$ mM; $[K^+]_o = 5$ mM; $[K^+]_i = 125$ mM; $P_{Na} = P_K$; and RT/F = 61.

Glutamate Has Several Ionotropic Receptors

Up to this point, we have focused on the nAChR because it has served as a model for the ionotropic receptor class, and an enormous amount of information is known about the behavior of this receptor-channel complex. However, several other ligand-specific ionotropic channels of great importance exist in the CNS. One set of receptors in this category include two types of glutamate receptor, the *NMDA receptor* and the non-NMDA receptors, *AMPA* and *kainate*, all of which are also cation-selective, fast-EPSP-producing receptors. The names for these receptor types stem from a pharmacological history: like the nAChR, so-called because it can be selectively activated by the "pharmacological" agent nicotine, the glutamate receptors in the ionotropic group derive their names from the pharmacological agents that serve as selective agonists of them. Thus the NMDA receptor is named for *N-methyl-D-aspartate*, the AMPA receptor for α-*amino*-3-hydroxy-5-*methyl*isoxazole-4-*propionic acid*, and the kainate receptor for kainate. The NMDA receptor is selectively blocked by the compound 2-*amino*-5-*phosphonovaleric* acid (APV); AMPA and kainate receptors are selectively blocked by 6-*cyano*-7-*nitroquinoxaline*-2,3-dione (CNQX). Numerous other agonists and antagonists of these receptors exist; and the receptors, like the nAChR, are formed by multimeric protein subunits (five for the NMDA receptor, probably three to four for AMPA and kainate receptors); and for each of these receptor types there are four to five subtypes composed of various subunit gene products that are differentially expressed in different cells. The subtypes of AMPA receptors are, in more recent classification schemes, based on gene families, designated as four different receptors, GluR1-4; kainate family members include GluR5-7 and KA1 and KA2; and ionotropic NMDA receptors as NR1 and NR2A to NR2D. Nonetheless, there is 50% to 80% homology among the various types and subtypes of ionotropic glutamate receptors, and all of these are (more distantly) related to the nAChR and to ionotropic receptors for the inhibitory transmitters glycine and γ-aminobutyric acid (GABA) as well.

Glutamate is the transmitter used by pyramidal cells of the cerebral cortex and by most primary sensory neurons (and other neurons as well), so receptors for this transmitter are widespread in the CNS and have formidable importance in brain function. Besides mediating many "routine" functions, such as initiating movements and processing incoming sensory information, these receptors are intimately involved in memory

and learning circuits, may well play a role in schizophrenia, and are certainly involved in responses to injury. The NMDA receptor, because it allows the entry of Ca^{++} ions into the cell (see below), can induce subsequent cellular events by calcium signaling, from activation of other functional intracellular metabolic pathways to causing cell death (referred to as *excitotoxicity*, since the death of the cell is caused by overstimulation by excitatory amino acids). The NMDA receptor has a unique feature that sets it apart from all other known ligand-gated channels. At the resting membrane potential, the opening of this channel is blocked by extracellular Mg^{2+} ions. Thus, even in the presence of glutamate, this channel permits little or no cation flux until the Mg^{2+} ions are displaced from the channel opening. The Mg^{2+} ions can only be removed from the channel opening if the transmembrane potential is depolarized—a depolarized (more positive) intracellular potential will cause displacement of the Mg^{2+} ions and then allow ion fluxes through the channel. This property of the NMDA receptor-channel makes it appear to be not only ligand gated but also voltage sensitive. In practical terms, the consequences of this property are that the NMDA channels will only open after the neuron has been depolarized by some other transmitter or by glutamate at its other receptor-channel complexes, such as the AMPA receptors. Another important feature of the NMDA receptor is that its ionophore channel is permeable to Ca^{2+}, as well as to Na^+ and K^+ ions. Thus Ca^{2+} influx normally accompanies opening of this channel. Finally, the NMDA receptor also has on its extracellular surface a binding site for the amino acid glycine. There is normally enough glycine circulating in the extracellular fluid that this site is occupied, but if glycine is not present, the receptor does not open in the presence of glutamate. The functional significance of the glycine binding is not yet clear. AMPA and NMDA receptors are often co-localized beneath a presynaptic

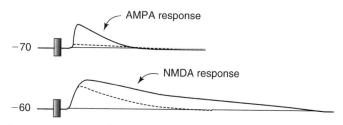

Figure 7-4 ■ Synaptic responses produced by glutamate at non-NMDA and NMDA receptors. The upper trace shows an EPSP produced in a neuron when glutamate interacts with an AMPA receptor at a normal resting potential. The EPSP is fast because of opening of cationic channels in AMPA receptors. If the AMPA receptors are blocked with CNQX, one might detect a very small NMDA receptor– induced response as indicated by the dotted line. Most of the NMDA channels are blocked at the resting potential by extracellular Mg++ ions. The lower trace is of the membrane potential from the same neuron, but now the cell is somewhat depolarized from rest because of summed inputs from AMPA (or other inputs). The depolarization has removed the Mg++ block from NMDA channels so that now when the same presynaptic glutamatergic input is stimulated, we see an EPSP that represents contributions from both the AMPA receptors and from the NMDA receptors. The dotted line in this trace represents the shape of the pure AMPA response that is now summed with the NMDA response; such an AMPA receptor–induced response would be seen if APV were added to block NMDA receptors. The EPSP in the lower trace is a somewhat larger and slightly more prolonged response than the pure AMPA response, and part of the inward current through the opened NMDA ionophore includes Ca++ ions.

glutamatergic terminal. Stimulation of the presynaptic glutamatergic axon releases glutamate that binds to both receptor types. However, since the NMDA receptor is blocked by Mg++ ions, only the response caused by the AMPA receptor is seen. The AMPA receptor produces a rapid and short-lived fast EPSP (Figure 7-4). Repeated stimulation permits summation of the AMPA responses and the induced depolarization removes the Mg++ block, and now the NMDA-induced currents can flow. The NMDA EPSP is a slightly slower and more long-lasting response that can, through Ca++ influx through the NMDA receptor ionophore, signal other events in the postsynaptic neuron.

Only a few other receptors of this class that produce fast, directly ligand-gated ionotropic EPSPs are well described—the 5-HT$_3$ receptor for serotonin and one substance K receptor.

Some Ionotropic Receptor Ionophores Are Selective for Cl⁻ or K⁺ and Cause Inhibition

There are, however, two important groups of this receptor-ionophore, fast PSP class that account for important inhibitory responses (IPSPs) in the CNS. One set is the *glycine receptor*, a multimeric protein complex (five subunits) that in the presence of bound glycine ligand opens a chloride-selective channel. This receptor is especially prominent in the brainstem and spinal cord. There are at least two isoforms of this receptor. Strychnine and picrotoxin are well-known pharmacological blockers of the channel, the former being a selective antagonist, the latter a noncompetitive inhibitor. The other fast IPSP receptor is the *GABA$_A$ receptor* (five subunits, molecularly closely related to the glycine receptor-channel and more distantly related to the glutamate receptor group; there are several subtypes of this receptor) also opens a chloride-selective channel. GABA is the major inhibitory transmitter in several brain regions, including the cerebellum, cerebral cortex, and striatum.

The $GABA_A$ receptor is especially interesting, and a few of its pharmacological features are discussed. It is also used to illustrate how post-synaptic inhibition operates. In addition to having two binding sites for GABA, the $GABA_A$ receptor also has binding sites for benzodiazepines (antianxiety agents such as diazepam [Valium]), barbiturates, and alcohol. These substances have allosteric actions on the receptor that can enhance its binding of GABA, and thus there is a logic for understanding how such compounds can have "inhibitory" (i.e., relaxing, sedative, or calming) effects and considerable clinical (and abuse) significance. This ionotropic receptor produces its inhibitory effect by increasing chloride conductance (Figure 7-5). The best-characterized pharmacological antagonist of this receptor is the compound bicuculline; muscimol is an effective agonist.

Mechanisms of Inhibition

In most neurons the equilibrium potential for chloride E_{Cl} is a few millivolts more negative than the resting membrane potential. For example, the resting potential may be –65 mV, and E_{Cl} –70 mV. If the $GABA_A$ receptor is activated by a puff of GABA, the chloride-selective ionotropic receptor will open and Cl^- ions will move through the channel in response to the electrochemical gradient acting on them. At the resting potential the inwardly directed concentration gradient for Cl^- slightly exceeds the outward electrical driving force on these negative ions (Figure 7-5, *A*). Opening the $GABA_A$ channel will result in an inward movement of Cl^- ions, and this will cause the membrane potential to move in the negative direction, away from threshold (Figure 7-5, *B*). It is less likely that the neuron can produce an action potential during this IPSP, so the cell is inhibited. If the membrane potential is moved to a more positive value using "current clamp" and GABA is added, the IPSP is larger. When the membrane potential is hyperpolarized to –70 mV, the addition of GABA causes no change in potential; at greater hyperpolarizations, application of GABA now generates a positive going potential change, an inverted or reversed IPSP. When the membrane potential is beyond (more negative) than –70 mV, the internal negativity creates a net outward electrical gradient that exceeds the inward concentration gradient for Cl^-, so Cl^- ions move *out* of the cell during the time the $GABA_A$ channel is open. A net outward movement of negative charge obviously allows the membrane potential to move in the positive direction. Because there was no potential change induced by GABA at –70 mV, it is assumed that no net current moved across the membrane. Thus –70 mV is the equilibrium potential for chloride. The reversal of the Cl^-–dependent IPSP at –70 mV is comparable to the reversal potential for ACh at –10 mV illustrated in Figure 7-2. It is the potential at which the transmitter-induced conductance increase causes no net movement of ions across the membrane. Of course, the case of chloride is simpler: only one ion is moving through the channel, so the reversal potential is the same as the equilibrium potential for that ion. In the case of cationic channels the reversal potential is determined by the contributions of increased conductance for both sodium and potassium, and since the increases in g_{Na} and g_K are equal, the reversal potential is equally situated between E_{Na} and E_K.

As discussed above, in most nerve cells E_{Cl} is somewhat more negative than the resting potential, so a glycine- or GABA-induced IPSP that occurs at the resting potential results in a net inward movement of Cl^- ions and a hyperpolarization that moves the membrane potential away from threshold. In some neurons, however, E_{Cl} lies between the resting potential and threshold. (This

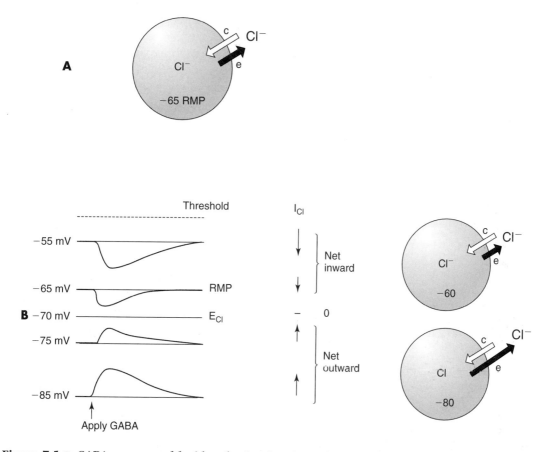

Figure 7-5 ■ GABA opens a chloride-selective fast ionophore. **A,** The circle represents a typical neuron with a resting potential of –65 mV. In such a cell, the inward concentration gradient (*open arrow* across the membrane) is slightly greater than the outward electrical gradient (*filled arrow*). **B,** A current clamp experiment in a neuron with GABA$_A$ receptors. When GABA is applied at the normal resting membrane potential (RMP, –65 mV), the GABA$_A$ ionophore opens and Cl$^-$ ions move into the cell, because at rest the net electrochemical gradient is inward for this ion. This causes an IPSP, and the cell is inhibited because the membrane potential is moved in the negative direction away from threshold. When the membrane potential is more depolarized by the current clamp (–55 mV), application of GABA produces a larger hyperpolarization because the outward electrical gradient is reduced and more net inward movement of Cl$^-$ ionic current occurs. If the neuron is hyperpolarized by injected current to –70 mV, there is no net movement of Cl$^-$ ions across the membrane and no GABA-induced potential change is seen. When the membrane is further hyper-polarized (–75 mV), the GABA-induced IPSP is seen to be inverted and becomes larger the more hyperpolarized the cell becomes (–85 mV). The inverted responses are caused by a net *outward* movement of Cl$^-$ ions because the imposed internal negativity creates an outward electrical gradient on these negative ions that exceeds the inward concentration gradient. In this case the reversal potential for this receptor is –70 mV, and this value of membrane potential also represents E$_{Cl}$.

is generally due to differences in intracellular chloride concentration produced by Cl^- pumps: a higher internal chloride ion concentration will reduce the concentration gradient on Cl^- ions and E_{Cl} will be more positive.) The resting potential might be -60 mV, E_{Cl} -55 mV, and threshold -50 mV. In these cells, when inhibitory transmitter is released, the cell, as always, moves toward E_{Cl} and the membrane potential goes in the *upward, positive* direction. There is a net *outward* movement of Cl^- ions. Although the membrane potential response to an increase in g_{Cl} is to move positive (toward threshold), the net effect of the response is still *inhibitory* because the increase in g_{Cl} means that the cell's potential will move to E_{Cl} but *not* beyond. Remember, the membrane potential moves to the equilibrium potential of the ion to which it is permeable. Thus it is as if the cell were voltage clamped at E_{Cl}, and the membrane potential cannot go any further toward threshold. The cell is effectively inhibited in that the cell cannot reach threshold. IPSPs caused by an increase in permeability to K^+ ions are always negative going, or hyperpolarizing, in a cell at the resting potential because E_K is always more negative than the resting potential.

One further important aspect of synaptic inhibition is the role played by the increase in conductance. The reduction in membrane resistance (i.e., the increase in conductance caused by inhibitory transmitters) is every bit as important, sometime more so, than the negative movement of membrane potential. This is explained by Ohm's law where $V = IR$, or, a potential change (V) can be produced by current (I) flowing through a resistor (R). An EPSP, for example, is a positive-going, depolarizing potential change (V) produced by a transmitter-induced flow of current (I) through the membrane resistance (R) of a neuron. If the membrane resistance of the cell were reduced in some way, then the excitatory synaptic current would produce a smaller poten-

tial change. An important way that IPSPs inhibit cells is that they, by increasing conductance to Cl^- or K^+, do decrease membrane resistance. If, during this period of reduced resistance, an EPSP were produced in the cell, its current would be less effective in depolarizing the cell. The EPSP would be smaller than normal and the cell would be less excited than it would have been if the IPSP had not occurred. It is as if the local, electrotonic currents produced with the EPSP were led away through the Cl^- or K^+ channels opened by the inhibitory transmitter. The EPSP, in complete analogy to an electrical circuit, is said to be shunted through a low-resistance pathway. Thus another form of inhibition can be a reduction in on-going excitatory events. The amplitude of EPSPs can also be modulated by other mechanisms called *presynaptic inhibition or facilitation*. These processes are described later.

■ QUESTIONS   *(Answers at end of the chapter)*

5. Discuss the unique property of the NMDA receptor.

6. How and why would the opening of K^+ channels in a resting neuron inhibit the cell?

7. If a neuron were voltage clamped at an internal potential of -40 mV and GABA was applied to the cell, explain what would happen to Cl^- ions and the membrane potential when $GABA_A$ receptors were activated.

■ METABOTROPIC RECEPTORS

Although the ionotropic receptors are numerous, potent, and important, they only represent a subset of receptor types found in the nervous system. The second great class of ligand-gated receptors is very different from those already described—different in their molecular structure, their mode of action, and the duration of their actions. Potential changes induced by these receptors can be, in contrast to those produced by ionotropic receptors, slower in onset and time-to-peak but are distinctively longer in duration, lasting for many tens of milliseconds to seconds, minutes, or hours. These receptors then produce *"slow"* EPSPs and IPSPs. This family of receptors is designated *metabotropic* receptors because they achieve their effects by secondary signaling through cascades of biochemical (metabolic) reactions in the cell. These receptor proteins do not form an ionophore in the membrane, but they affect ion channels elsewhere in the membrane *indirectly* through these biochemical reactions and so-called *second messengers*. ("Second messenger" was coined to distinguish these molecules from the "first" or "primary" messenger, the synaptic transmitter itself.)

Metabotropic Receptors Share a Common Molecular Design and Function through Complex Biochemical Pathways

Metabotropic receptors are composed of a single, large protein that has seven membrane-spanning regions (the protein is not multimeric) (Figure 7-6). There is considerable homology among the receptors of this family, and all are related to rhodopsin and possibly descended from an ancient molecule similar to bacteriorhodopsin, but there is vast diversity among the extant receptors known today. The large *N*-terminal extracellular stretch of the protein is glycosylated and is the recognition/binding site for polypeptides and proteins. The binding site for small-molecule transmitters, such as noradrenalin (norepinephrine) or ACh, is located on parts of the molecule associated with loops of the transmembrane helices deep in the outer edge of the membrane. The receptors interact with membrane-associated (intracellular) proteins, namely the so-called G-proteins ("G" because of their affinity for GTP/GDP). This family of receptors is also designated as the *G-protein-coupled receptor class*. The G-protein binding area is located on one or more intracellular loops of the receptor protein (Figure 7-6, *A*). The intracellular carboxy-terminal part of the receptor protein has serine phosphorylation sites, which when phosphorylated can alter the activity of the receptor.

The G-protein is partially imbedded in the inner leaflet of the cell membrane, lying close to metabotropic receptors. This is a trimeric protein with three subunits (Figure 7-6, *B*). Two of these, the β and γ subunits, are tightly bound to one another and function as a unit. This dimer links G-protein to the membrane inner leaflet. The third subunit, α, is loosely bound to the βγ subunit and it also has the binding site for the guanine nucleotides. In the absence of transmitter, the trimeric G-protein complex is bound together and linked to GDP through the α subunit. When the appropriate transmitter binds to the receptor, it induces a conformational change that permits the G-protein-binding loop to bind to the α subunit that actually moves laterally in the membrane to associate with the receptor. This allows the α subunit to exchange the GDP for GTP; the βγ subunit is required for this reaction. The α-subunit-GTP complex is now able to bind to yet another protein, called generically a *primary effector protein*, which is an enzyme located nearby in association with the membrane. The activated effector molecule then catalyzes the production of second messenger molecules to carry out a variety of specific activities in the cell. Most of the second messengers in turn activate other enzymes (*secondary effectors*) that induce biochemical events and products that can influence a variety of cellular events, including effects on ion channels. Most of these secondary effectors are protein kinases that phosphorylate other proteins, such as channel proteins. Ion channels that are opened (or closed) by this process can be either the familiar voltage-gated channels, or they can be other

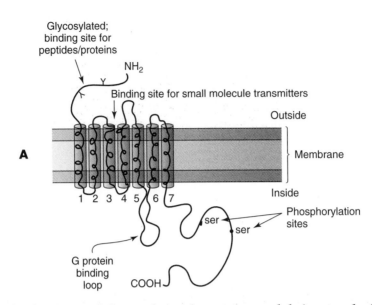

Figure 7-6 ■ Molecular nature of the metabotropic receptors and their general relationship to other membrane-associated signaling molecules A, Metabotropic receptors consist of one large protein that has seven membrane-spanning α-helices. On the extracellular surface the *N*-terminal domain is glycosylated and has binding sites for proteins. Small-molecule transmitters bind in a region of the molecule formed by loops of the α-helices between transmembrane domains 3 and 4. This binding site is rather deep within the outer edge of the lipid bilayer of the membrane. The intracellular C-terminal portion of the receptor has serine residues that can be phosphorylated. An intracellular loop between transmembrane segments 5 and 6 serves as the major binding domain for G-proteins. This loop may also have serine or threonine residues that can be phosphorylated.

Ligand + Receptor→G-Protein→Effector Protein→Second Messengers→Secondary Effector→Channels

↑ αβγ   ↑ α-GTP   (enzymes)   ↑ catalysis   (often kinases) ↑   open, close

channels that underlie slow EPSPs and IPSPs. Although this is complicated, the illustration above is a general scheme that applies to the functional organization of all of the metabotropic receptor responses.

The real complexity, diversity, and flexibility of this system derives from the fact that the different elements of the scheme are combined in different ways in different cells, so that a receptor of one type can be linked to different G-

proteins in different cells. Of course, there are many different types of all the players. There are many different transmitter ligands, and all of these have multiple subtypes of receptor. Virtually all of the transmitters mentioned with respect to ionotropic receptors, such as acetylcholine, glutamate, and GABA; a large number of peptide transmitters; ATP and adenosine; and the biogenic amines (noradrenalin, adrenalin, dopamine, serotonin, histamine) have receptors in the meta-

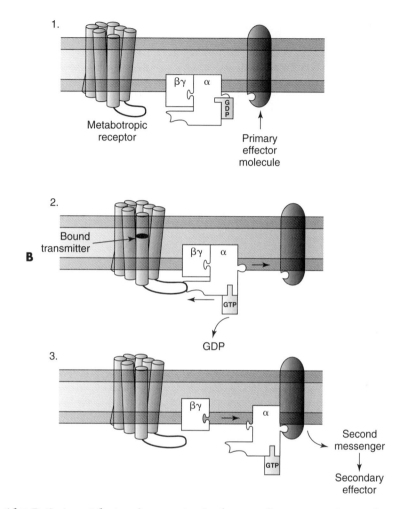

Figure 7-6 cont'd ■ B, *1*, A metabotropic receptor is shown adjacent to a G-protein. G-proteins are trimeric with 3 subunits, α, β, and γ. The β and γ subunits are tightly bound to one another and anchor the complex in the membrane. The α subunit has a guanosine binding site. In an unactivated G-protein, the α subunit is bound to GDP. Near the receptor and G-protein are other membrane-associated molecules called *primary effector molecules.* These are typically enzymes. B, *2*, When a transmitter binds to the metabotropic receptor, a conformational change is induced so that the receptor binds to the α subunit of the G-protein via the loop described above. This triggers the βγ dimer subunit to assist the α subunit to exchange GDP for GTP, and the α subunit dissociates from the complex. B, *3*, This now permits the α subunit to bind to the primary effector molecular, activating that enzyme, which is then able to catalyze the production of second messenger molecules that can influence other effector molecules, biochemical processes, or ion channel properties.

TABLE 7-1

TABLE 7-1

Some Metabotropic Receptors and Associated G-Proteins*

Receptor	G-protein	Receptor	G-protein
mAChR		**Dopamine**	
M1, M3, M5	$G_{i/o}$	D1, D5	G_s
M2, M4	G_q	D2–D4	$G_{i/o}$
GABA$_B$		**Serotonin**	
R_{1a}, R_{1b}, R_2	G_I	5-HT$_{1A-1E}$	$G_{i/o}$
		5-HT$_{2A-2C}$	G_q
Glutamate		5-HT$_{4-7}$	G_s
Group I: mGluR1 and mGluR2	G_q	**Histamine**	
Groups II and III: mGluR2-5	G_I	H1	G_q
		H2	G_s
Adrenalin/noradrenalin		H3	?
(epinephrine/norepinephrine)			
		ATP, adenosine	
$\alpha_{1A, 1B, 1C}$	G_q	P$_1$:A$_1$ and A$_3$	$G_{i/o}$
$\alpha_{2A, 2B, 2C}$	$G_{i/o}$	A$_{2A}$, A$_{2B}$	G_s
$\beta_{1 \text{ and }} \beta_2$	G_s	P$_{2Y}$'s	G_q, $G_{i/o}$
β_3	$\alpha_s/G_{i/o}$		

*Most of the metabotropic receptor subtypes for the small-molecule transmitters are shown with the G-protein on which they act. The list is simplified, and G-protein subunits can have multiple actions. The terminology for differentiating G-proteins is in constant flux. The first G-protein discovered *stimulated* adenylyl cyclase, so was named G_s. Then G-proteins that *inhibited* adenylyl cyclase were described as G_i. Newer ones were initially designated G_o for *other* kinds of effects, but this subset has been further expanded and G-proteins with specific actions renamed. G-proteins acting on PLC were first called G_p-proteins but are now usually designated G_q-proteins. New subtypes are being characterized or cloned, so the terminology is likely to continue to evolve.

botropic class. All of these transmitters have several receptor subtypes (Table 7-1). Furthermore, the receptors have varying selectivity for the transmitters and differing pharmacological profiles. The properties of the receptors (e.g., their affinity for ligand) can be influenced by allosteric effects of other chemicals and by whether or not the receptor is phosphorylated.

The next level of complexity arises from the fact that there are several different α subunits of the G-proteins that can have various effects on the primary effector molecules, serving to activate (stimulate) them, to inhibit them, or to

have other effects on their activity. In fact, α subunits are typically designated by a subscript that specifies the type of action they produce on certain effector enzymes or for the effector itself: α_s indicates α subunits that stimulate adenylyl cyclase; α_i, subunits that inhibit that effector; α_q for subunits that act on phospholipase C; and probably 20 or more other forms of this subunit exist. (Usually, the entire G-protein is named for the action of its α subunit; thus there are families of G_s, G_i, G_q, G_o (and so on) proteins; see Table 7-1.) The G-proteins have been isolated and functionally characterized by a variety of biochemical, gene-cloning, and functional studies. Important insights into their activity were in part derived by research that showed that the physiological effects of certain bacterial toxins were mediated by their effects on α subunits. Cholera toxin, for example, irreversibly activates certain α_s subunits by inhibiting their GTPase activity. Inability to hydrolyze GTP will prevent the α_s subunit from dissociating with its primary effector molecule, and this results in sustained, nonphysiological activity in the pathway. Pertussis toxin, however, inactivates certain α subunits, preventing them from activating the appropriate effector molecules.

■ **QUESTIONS**   *(Answers at end of the chapter)*

8. Describe the major structural features of metabotropic receptors.

9. Discuss how G-proteins function as "transducers" of molecular information.

This large variety of G-proteins then can act on several primary effector proteins that catalyze production of different second messenger molecules (Figure 7-7). The best understood primary effector molecules are the following:

1. Adenylyl cyclase catalyzes the formation of cyclic adenosine monophosphate (cAMP, the second messenger) that can then act on cAMP-dependent kinases (usually protein kinase A [PKA], a secondary effector) that can phosphorylate other molecules, including ion channels, to open or close them.

2. Phospholipase C (PLC) hydrolyzes a membrane-bound phospholipid, phosphatidylinositol 4,5-biphosphate (PIP_2), into inositol-tri-phosphate (IP_3) and diacylglycerolphosphate (DAG). The IP_3 is soluble in the cytosol and reacts with membranes of the endoplasmic reticulum to release Ca^{++} from intracellular stores; the increased Ca^{++} levels can have multiple effects on other biochemical processes and on the behavior of certain ion channels. Ca^{++} itself can also act as a second messenger. One of its possible actions is to interact with a small protein molecule called calmodulin; the Ca^{++}-calmodulin complex then reacts with another protein kinase, Ca^{++}-calmodulin–dependent kinase (CaM-kinase), which by phosphorylation can modulate channels. The DAG product of PIP_2 hydrolysis remains in the membrane and activates protein kinase C (PKC), which can phosphorylate many different intracellular proteins.

3. Phospholipase A_2, a primary effector molecule, triggers, via hydrolysis of phosphatidylinositol (PI), the production of arachidonic acid (second messenger) that in turn is metabolized into numerous biologically active compounds, such as prostaglandins and other metabolites, some of which also can modulate channels. There is considerable heterogeneity and variability in these pathways and in the uses or roles of various of the molecular players. For example, sometimes the βγ subunit activates an effector or a channel, and some second messengers can directly affect channels or other proteins in addition to their ability to activate kinases.

Further regulation occurs by additional sets of enzymes. The second messengers, cAMP and cyclic guanosine 3′-5′ monophosphate (cGMP) are broken down by phosphodiesterase enzymes whose activity is highly regulated. Similarly, there are many phosphatase enzymes that dephosphorylate various proteins, including channel proteins, which have been phosphorylated by the secondary effector kinases. The phosphatases too are regulated and critical for terminating many transmitter-induced events.

The complexity of these systems and their possible sites of interaction are truly extraordinary (Figure 7-8), and new details are being filled in on a continuous basis. Nonetheless, it is already clear that the biochemical characteristics of these complex pathways impose three qualities to the

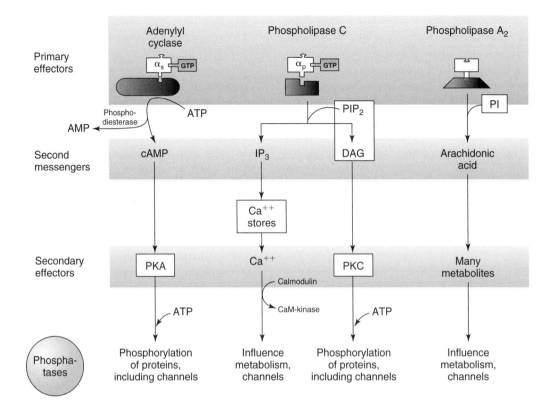

Figure 7-7 ■ **The three major biochemical signaling pathways that metabotropic receptors can activate. The three primary effector enzyme proteins activated by metabotropic receptors via G-proteins are illustrated. These are adenylyl cyclase, phospholipase C, and phospholipase A$_2$. Each of these effectors then produces second messenger molecules: cAMP, IP$_3$ and DAG, and arachidonic acid, respectively. These compounds can then induce activity in so-called secondary effectors, including protein kinases or other biochemical agents, or can cause increases in intracellular Ca^{++} levels. These secondary effectors, often via phosphorylation of downstream proteins, can alter ion channels (ligand- and voltage-gated channels), induce a variety of biochemical events, or induce gene transcription. The boxes drawn around PIP$_2$, DAG, and PI indicate that these molecules are attached to the inner leaflet of the membrane. The circle of phosphatases at the lower left represents this family of highly regulated enzymes that can dephosphorylate the various protein phosphorylated by the kinases. Some second messengers, such as cAMP and Ca^{++} ions, can also directly influence channels, regulate other enzymes, or influence transmitter release. Ca^{++} ions also influence cell processes by binding to calmodulin and inducing CaM-kinases.**

responses produced by this group of receptors: (1) the effects of these receptors can be relatively slow to develop since sequential cascades of events follow receptor activation, and the respons-es are long lasting, persisting for seconds to minutes to hours or longer; (2) there is an amplification phenomenon that accompanies these responses: a few activated receptors can activate

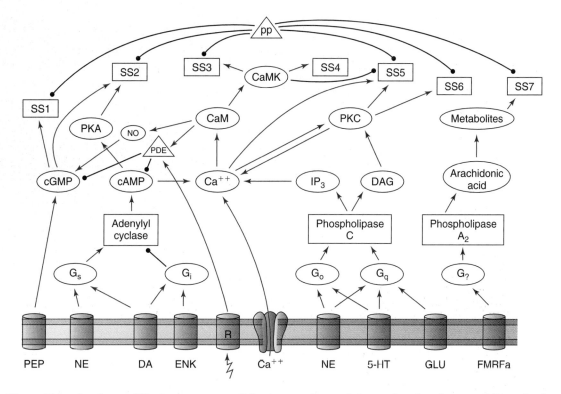

Figure 7-8 ■ **A schema illustrating some of the interactions of the molecules that participate in the biochemical cascades that are induced by metabotropic receptors. At the bottom are shown several representative types of metabotropic receptors:** *PEP,* **a receptor for certain peptides that can lead to an increase in production of cGMP;** *NE,* **a norepinephrine receptor that activates G_s, which then activates adenylyl cyclase;** *DA,* **a dopamine receptor that activates G_i, which can inhibit adenylyl cyclase;** *ENK,* **an encephalin (another peptide) receptor that activates G_i;** *R,* **a rhodopsin molecule whose activation by light (***jagged arrow***) can activate phosphodiesterases; Ca^{++}, a voltage-gated Ca^{++} channel, of which there are several (or other sources of transmembrane Ca^{++}, such as ionotropic NMDA receptors);** *NE,* **another norepinephrine receptor that activates other G proteins (G_o or G_q); 5-HT, a serotonin receptor that activates G_o or G_q; a glutamate** *(GLU)* **receptor that activates G_q;** *FMRFa,* **a receptor for this peptide that works through uncertain G-protein intermediates to activate phospholipase A_2. Subsets of G_o and G_q can activate phospholipase C (PLC). Ca^{++} ions, arachidonic acid and its metabolites, and the products of adenylyl cyclase and PLC activities, including cAMP, IP_3, and DAG, act as second messengers. Typically, these activate phosphokinases (PKA, PKC, and CaMK), but most also have the capability for direct effects on many other metabolic pathways or protein activities. The kinases can phosphorylate proteins, including ion channels. SS1–SS7 represent varieties of substrate proteins on which second messengers and kinases might act (ion channel proteins, regulators of gene transcription, enzymes, proteins regulating release of transmitter, etc). Phosphodiesterases** *(PDE; triangle)* **hydrolyze cGMP and cAMP; phosphatases** *(PP, triangle)* **dephosphorylate proteins whose activities were altered by kinase-induced phosphorylation.** *NO,* **Nitric oxide. Lines with arrows indicate stimulation or activation; lines with filled circles indicate inhibition.** (Modified from Kennedy MB: Second messengers and neuronal function. In Hall ZW (ed): *An introduction to molecular neurobiology,* Sunderland, Mass, 1992, Sinauer Associates, pp 207–246.)

many more G-proteins, these in turn can initiate multiple cycles of primary effector activation, and the primary effectors—often enzymes—can catalyze the production of many second messengers; and (3) since most second messenger molecules, or their target enzymes or target-enzyme products, are freely soluble in the cytosol, a single receptor can influence the behavior of cell processes and channel states over a wide expanse of membrane. Indeed, the types of slow, relatively small, and persistent synaptic responses produced by these receptors are sometimes referred to as *modulatory* responses.

■ **QUESTIONS** *(Answers at end of the chapter)*

10. Name the enzyme that catalyzes the production of each of the following second messengers: cAMP, IP_3, DAG, and arachidonic acid.

11. Name at least one action that each of the same second messengers and Ca^{++} ions can have in a neuron.

12. Name two more things Ca^{++} ions can do.

Some Physiological Effects of Metabotropic Receptor Activation

To better appreciate the way this complex biochemical and molecular machinery operates, we will examine a few examples of specific metabotropic receptors. Some of these are involved in the production of slow PSPs, and others regulate voltage-gated channels or other processes in the cell. Probably the most thoroughly characterized of the metabotropic receptors is the β-adrenergic receptor (βAR) and its cAMP second messenger pathway. When noradrenalin (norepinephrine) binds to the $β_1AR$ in heart muscle, a stimulatory $α_s$ subunit of the G-protein activates adenylyl cyclase and cAMP is produced, which then activates protein kinase A (PKA). In the heart, the PKA phosphorylates and

activates L-type voltage-gated Ca^{++} channels. This in turn causes an increase in the Ca^{++}-dependent action potential plateau of cardiac fibers and the well-known increase in force and rate of heart muscle contraction caused by noradrenalin (or adrenalin or agonists of these transmitters, such as isoproterenol). In pyramidal neurons in the cerebral cortex, other β-adrenergic receptors may act by blocking Ca^{++}-dependent K^+ channels, which by slowing action potential repolarization and thus prolonging the period of depolarization could contribute to increased excitability of these neurons.

Many of the large variety of noradrenergic and adrenergic receptor types, such as the $β_1AR$ mentioned in the heart, and others in the α-adrenergic receptor class, are expressed in the autonomic nervous system and target tissues of postganglionic autonomic neurons. An important metabotropic receptor for acetylcholine has also been characterized in autonomic ganglia. Metabotropic ACh receptors are also called muscarinic ACh receptors (mAChRs), in analogy to ionotropic nAChRs, because an alkaloid, muscarine, isolated from certain mushrooms, is a pharmacological agonist for most of these receptors. Another alkaloid, atropine, derived from the belladonna plant, is a widely used antagonist of muscarinic receptors. The muscarinic receptor in postganglionic autonomic neurons produces a slow EPSP and allows us to contrast a slow EPSP with a fast one. If one stimulates a preganglionic autonomic neuron, it releases ACh onto postganglionic neurons. The response of certain postganglionic cells comprises at least two different EPSPs (Figure 7-9). The first is a rapid depolarizing event caused by nAChRs on the postganglionic neuron. This first, fast EPSP is followed a bit later by a smaller and more long-lasting (few seconds) depolarizing response. This second, slow EPSP is caused by mAChRs (of the M1, M3, M5 group), and it is generated by *closing* special K^+ channels called the M-type (for muscarinic) that are nor-

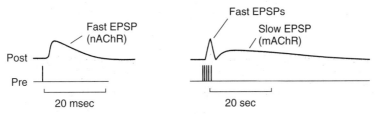

Figure 7-9 ■ Fast and slow EPSPs can be recorded in certain postganglionic neurons in the autonomic nervous system. *Left,* A single stimulus to a preganglionic axon *(Pre)* produces a brisk EPSP in the postganglionic cell *(Post).* This response can be mimicked by exogenously applied ACh and nicotine and is blocked by curare. It is produced by nAChR and is completed in 20–30 msec. *Right,* Repetitive stimulation of the presynaptic axon produces the summated fast EPSP and is followed by a different EPSP, one that has a longer latency, smaller amplitude, and dramatically longer time course (note the compressed time for the traces on the right). This slow EPSP can also be mimicked by ACh and by muscarinic (not nicotinic) agonists, and the response can be blocked by atropine (but not curare). The fast EPSP is caused by the opening of a cationic channel; the slow EPSP is caused by the closure of M-type K⁺ channels (see text).

mally open and contributing to the resting potassium conductance of unstimulated postganglionic neurons. The mAChR is a G-protein–coupled receptor, but the second messenger for this effect is uncertain; the receptor may activate phospholipase C via $G_{q/11}$ with subsequent increases in IP_3 and Ca^{++} concentrations and in DAG activity, but the exact linkage to K^+ channel proteins is not clear.

We can understand how closing of open K^+ channels could produce a depolarization by recalling that even at rest there are some open Na^+ channels (see Chapter 2); there is a small resting conductance for Na^+. If we reduce some of the K^+ conductance, the Na^+ conductance is now somewhat "unopposed," and the membrane potential will drift positively toward E_{Na}. Such slow EPSPs caused by a reduced conductance to K^+ ions are actually excitatory for two reasons. First, they obviously move the membrane potential nearer threshold. But second, since they are produced by a *decrease* in conductance, the membrane resistance of the cell is actually *increased.* In analogy to the earlier discussion of

the ability of inhibitory Cl^- and K^+ conductance increases to shunt excitatory inputs, now in these cells the higher resistance of the membrane during the slow EPSP will make other excitatory inputs *larger* than normal because their synaptic currents are flowing through a higher R_m.

As mentioned earlier, not all metabotropic responses depend on the full pathway from receptor to kinase-phosphorylated proteins. In the heart, for example, a G-protein βγ subunit activated by an acetylcholine muscarinic receptor (M2, M4) is known to *directly* open a K^+ channel called the *G-protein–regulated inward rectifying K^+ (GIRK) channel.* Opening the channel hyperpolarizes heart pacemaker cells and slows the heartbeat. This is a "direct" pathway from G-protein to channel, bypassing intermediates such as second messengers or kinases. Second messengers, such as cAMP, can also directly modify channels. In photoreceptors of the retina, for example, another second messenger molecule, cGMP acts directly on sodium channels to open them and functions in this way in the dark. In the light,

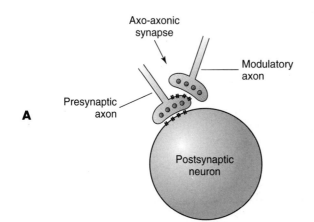

A

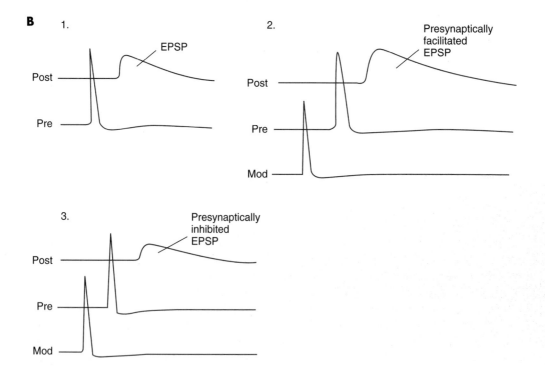

Figure 7-10 ■ For legend see opposite page.

Figure 7-10 ■ **Axo-axonic synapses underlie forms of presynaptic facilitation and inhibition.** A, Drawing of a synaptic arrangement with a presynaptic axon terminal making a conventional synapse onto a postsynaptic cell. Another axon labeled "modulatory" makes an axo-axonic synapse onto the presynaptic axon terminal. If an action potential invades the terminal of the presynaptic axon, a conventional EPSP is produced in the postsynaptic neuron (B, *1*). Firing the modulatory axon to precede the presynaptic action potential results in a larger, "facilitated" EPSP (B, *2*). The process is called *presynaptic facilitation.* In this example, modeled on the *Aplysia* sensory-to-motor synapse, the modulatory axon released the transmitter serotonin onto the presynaptic terminal. The 5-HT receptors there induced, via cAMP, a closing of potassium channels. This slowed repolarization of the presynaptic action potential, which allowed more Ca^{++} to enter the presynaptic terminal. The enhanced entry of Ca^{++} triggered additional transmitter release from the presynaptic terminal, thus generating a larger EPSP in the postsynaptic cell. Other axo-axonic synapses can cause the opposite effect (B, *3*), called *presynaptic inhibition.* In this case the modulatory axon's transmitter can activate processes in the presynaptic terminal that reduce the amount of transmitter released from the presynaptic axon. This results in a smaller than normal EPSP in the postsynaptic cell.

---

photons activate rhodopsin (structurally similar to metabotropic receptors), which then excites cGMP-phosphodiesterase. The phosphodiesterase breaks down the cGMP, and the Na^+ channels close.

A final example of metabotropic receptor actions is drawn from work on a well-known model preparation, the marine mollusk *Aplysia* (Figure 7-10). Certain sensory neurons in these animals receive inputs from other neurons that use serotonin (5-hydroxytryptamine, 5-HT) as their transmitter. The sensory cells have a metabotropic 5-HT receptor that is linked to the cAMP pathway and then to PKA. Application of 5-HT causes a slow EPSP in the sensory neurons that is believed to be due to the closing of a unique K^+ channel called the *S-type channel.* PKA-mediated phosphorylation of the channel protein can account for the channel closing. Closing of the channels allows the action potential in these neurons to be slightly prolonged. This allows more Ca^{++} to enter the terminal and more transmitter to be released from sensory neurons to their postsynaptic motoneurons— a form of synaptic modulation. In these same sensory cells, a peptide transmitter called

FMRFamide (containing the amino acids Phe-Met-Arg-Phe-amide) acts through a different metabotropic receptor to stimulate phospholipase A_2, which generates arachidonic acid. Certain downstream metabolites of arachidonic acid act on the same S-type K^+ channels to open them and thus hyperpolarize the sensory neurons.

It is important to appreciate that the responses produced by this large family of receptors can affect not only ionic channels in the membrane but also can have many other effects that do not change membrane conductance but instead alter cell metabolism, gene expression, or other biochemical processes (such as the transmitter-release process itself), some of which can influence channel expression or cell function over long-time scales. In the *Aplysia* sensory neurons mentioned previously, for example, repeated stimulation of the 5-HT receptors leads to increased amounts of PKA, which then can initiate other molecular events that induce gene transcription and the synthesis of new proteins that can sustain the enhanced synaptic response in motoneurons for weeks, even build new synapses and more active zones.

■ **QUESTIONS**   *(Answers at end of the chapter)*

13. If an appropriate amount of atropine were added to the autonomic ganglion preparation as discussed with Figure 7-9, how would this influence the recordings shown in the right-hand panel of that figure?

14. Discuss why changing the membrane resistance of a neuron could have an influence on PSPs.

15. Why does turning off potassium conductance depolarize a cell?

■ **PRESYNAPTIC FACILITATION AND INHIBITION**

The 5-HT receptors on the *Aplysia* sensory cells are found in the axon terminals of these neurons where the serotonin-containing interneurons send their axon terminals to form axo-axonic synapses with the sensory endings. Such axo-axonic synapses are widespread in all nervous systems and represent an important function carried out by nerve cells, namely, modulation of the amount of transmitter that can be released from one synaptic terminal by another synaptic ending. One nerve cell axon ends on another nerve cell's axon terminal. The terminology can get confusing here, so we will call the axon forming the original synapse on a postsynaptic cell the "presynaptic" axon (Figure 7-10). The axon ending on the presynaptic axon is called the "modulatory" axon (which is presynaptic to the "presynaptic" axon). Release of transmitter from the "modulatory axon" can activate receptors (ionotropic or metabotropic) on the "presynaptic" axon. These receptors can then influence the release of transmitter from the "presynaptic" axon onto its own postsynaptic follower cell. In the case of the *Aplysia* sensory neurons, serotonin from the "modulatory" axon terminal closed the S-type K^+ channel in the sensory neuron terminal

that allowed the action potential in the "presynaptic" sensory neuron to be prolonged. This provided more time for Ca^{++} ions to enter the presynaptic terminal, enhancing release of transmitter from the sensory ending so the postsynaptic EPSP in the motoneuron became larger. Thus a transmitter from one axon caused a change in function of another axon whose influence on its own follower cell was modified. From the "perspective" of the motoneuron, the EPSP it received from the sensory cell was enhanced. When a PSP in a neuron is enhanced in this way, the process is defined as *presynaptic facilitation*. (This is sometimes also called *heterosynaptic facilitation*, indicating that two *different* axons participated in causing the facilitation. This terminology differentiates this form of PSP enhancement from enhancement that might occur if the "presynaptic" terminal increased its transmitter release by some intrinsic process that did not involve input from another axon. An example of this kind of "independent" increase in transmitter release would be the phenomenon known as *post-tetanic potentiation*. Here, intense, repetitive stimulation of an axon can cause a change in the terminal, linked to a prolonged increase in Ca^{++}, so that shortly after the tetanus, single stimulations produce larger PSPs than the normal PSPs evoked before the stimulus train. This enhancement subsides over minutes but does represent a kind of *postsynaptic facilitation* that can occur involving a single synapse. Facilitatory events that are intrinsic to a single presynaptic axon are also sometimes called *homosynaptic facilitation*, meaning the same axon [and only that one] was involved in the facilitation.) Presynaptic facilitation occurs at other synapses, where it is believed that either nAChRs or kainate receptors may be activated in the "presynaptic" terminal, causing enough depolarization to turn on voltage-gated Ca^{++} channels and again enhance transmitter release.

The amount of transmitter released from a

terminal can also be *decreased* in a comparable process called *presynaptic inhibition*. Here, a "modulatory" axon releases a transmitter that produces a lessening of transmitter release from a "presynaptic" terminal, and thus a decrease in the EPSP in the postsynaptic neuron. Presynaptic inhibition could be caused by at least two different mechanisms. In one form, $GABA_A$ receptors in the "presynaptic" terminal could be activated by release of GABA from the "modulatory" axon terminal. If Cl^- conductance is high when an action potential invades the "presynaptic" terminal, part of the action potential current could be short-circuited, or shunted, through open Cl^- channels, causing a reduction in action potential height, less calcium entry, and less transmitter release. This mechanism applies regardless of whether E_{Cl} is at membrane more or less polarized than the resting potential (see previous section on Mechanisms of Inhibition). Presynaptic inhibition is also known to occur because certain metabotropic receptors in the presynaptic terminal lead to the closure of Ca^{++} channels and opening of K^+ channels, reducing calcium influx and shortening the spike. This also will reduce the amount of transmitter released, and the size of the postsynaptic EPSP will be smaller. It is also likely that presynaptic inhibition is produced in other terminals via metabotropic receptors whose secondarily activated products may interfere with the molecular machinery of release. EPSPs can be reduced by a homosynaptic process where the presynaptic axon, through intrinsic mechanisms, releases less transmitter with repetitive stimulation. This type of postsynaptic inhibition is sometimes called *habituation*.

Many axon terminals in the central nervous system have receptors on their surface for the transmitter that the terminal releases. These are called *autoreceptors*. They are metabotropic receptors that serve to modulate release of the transmitter from the terminal. Examples of these are the α_2 receptor at adrenergic terminals, the D_2

receptor at dopamine terminals, the $GABA_B$ receptor at GABA terminals, and the $5\text{-}HT_{1a}$ receptor at serotonergic terminals. Most of these receptors are linked to the G_i family of G-proteins and typically serve to reduce transmitter release by one of several mechanisms, including inhibition of voltage-gated Ca^{++} channels, activation of K^+ channels, or inhibition of adenylyl cyclase with consequent modulation of the release process.

■ QUESTIONS   *(Answers at the end of the chapter)*

16. Discuss in general terms the structure and physiology of the neural organization underlying presynaptic inhibition.

■ DESENSITIZATION

Another means by which synaptic efficacy can be changed is by a process called receptor *desensitization*. First described at the neuromuscular junction, desensitization was named for the observation that prolonged exposure to ACh made additional or subsequent applications of the transmitter less effective. If, for example, a blocker of acetylcholinesterase, such as the compound eserine (or physostigmine), was added to a preparation, this prevented the breakdown of ACh, and the transmitter remained in the vicinity of the receptors in higher concentrations. Stimulation of the motor axon under these conditions produced smaller than normal EPPs. It appeared that if receptors were exposed to "too much" transmitter, they stopped responding to it, or became desensitized. Desensitization has since been observed at many different synapses, and although its functional significance is not entirely understood, it may serve as a means of curtailing responsiveness if overstimulation of a synapse occurs. Studies at both cholinergic and adrenergic synapses have shown that at least two mechanisms exist for producing desensitization. One is relatively rapid, occurring within seconds to minutes, and is produced by phosphorylation of the receptor via PKA, PKC, or other kinases.

This can occur on certain of the subunits of ionotropic receptors or on cytoplasmic loops of metabotropic receptors; phosphorylation changes the receptor conformation so that it can no longer bind to ligand. The other means by which desensitization occurs is by sequestration and internalization of receptor, a process that make take hours to occur. Phosphorylation may also be involved, and participation of other proteins, such as clathrin and another protein called arrestin, appear to be required to actually endocytose the receptor. By reducing the number of receptors available to bind to transmitter, the postsynaptic cell's response to applied ligands may be reduced.

■ SOME "UNCONVENTIONAL" TRANS-SYNAPTIC MESSENGERS

The gas nitric oxide (NO) was first shown to be a signaling molecule in vascular tissue. Cholinergic autonomic input to endothelial cells in peripheral arteries was shown to induce the release from endothelial cells of this unexpected compound, which then moved into vascular smooth muscle fibers, causing them to relax. NO is highly soluble in lipids so it easily can move across membranes, requiring no special release or exocytosic process. NO has now been shown to be an intercellular messenger between neurons. Nitric oxide is produced by oxidation of the amino acid arginine by the enzyme NO synthase (NOS). NOS is a highly regulated enzyme; it is activated in neurons in the hippocampal cortex by glutamatergic inputs that activate NMDA receptors. Ca^{++} that enters the cell binds to calmodulin and the Ca^{++}-calmodulin complex activates NOS. Newly formed NO leaves the neuron and readily dissolves through the membrane of the presynaptic glutamatergic terminal. There it interacts with a cytosolic guanylyl cyclase to enhance the production of cGMP. This second messenger then induces an increase in glutamate transmitter release from the presynaptic terminal. It is believed that this NO "circuitry" may be the mechanism for producing the enhancement of synaptic transmission that accompanies some forms of learning and memory. There is increasing evidence that carbon monoxide may also act as an intercellular messenger in a manner comparable to NO. The discovery of gaseous agents with such properties have confounded our traditional view of synaptic transmission. NO is not stored in vesicles or released in packets by exocytosis; there is no conventional receptor in the membrane of the target cell—NO just passes through the membrane and stimulates the production of cGMP; there is no special uptake system or degradative pathway for NO. After being synthesized it remains in the vicinity of the synapses only for several seconds and then dissolves away into the bloodstream or decays into nitrite. Finally, based on its apparent actions in the nervous system as known to date, NO does not follow the rule about dynamic polarity of synapses and neuronal functional organization: instead of the message going from presynaptic to postsynaptic cell, it is going "backward." But there is logic to this scheme. Both the localization and activity of NOS and cGMP are tightly regulated in the brain, and neurobiologists have long theorized that to make learning happen via enhanced transmission at specific synapses, it makes sense for the postsynaptic cell to inform the presynaptic cell about the state of the postsynaptic neuron, or for the postsynaptic neuron to have a role in reinforcing the enhancement. It will be a remarkable irony if the basis for one of the most profound of all nervous events, the formation of abiding memories, resides in an ephemeral, transient molecule of gas.

■ IT IS THE RECEPTOR THAT COUNTS

There are many different receptor subtypes for the same transmitter. The specific effects produced by a transmitter (whether opening or closing ion channels, whether the channels are selective for ions that produce IPSPs or EPSPs, or whether the channels are voltage gated, whether the receptors are of the ionotropic or metabotropic type, what G protein subunits are involved, which effectors and second messengers are used, or whether other metabolic events are altered or gene transcription induced) *depend on the receptor*. Thus knowing what transmitter is used at a synapse is not enough to predict the effects of the transmitter because the same transmitter can have dramatically different effects depending on which receptor it activates. The critical element in the synaptic transmission equation is the receptor, not the transmitter. To say simply that acetylcholine is the transmitter at a particular synapse does not explain very much.

■ POST-TEST

1. The GABA$_B$ autoreceptor on GABAergic nerve terminals can actually cause a reduction in inhibition in the postsynaptic cell to which the terminal is functionally connected. How could this work?

2. If voltage-gated K$^+$ currents involved in action potential repolarization were blocked by actions of a metabotropic receptor, how would this change the action potential, and what important outcome might this have on transmitter release from the cell in which the channels were blocked?

3. Walk through the pathway from activation of an NMDA receptor in a postsynaptic cell to enhanced transmitter release from the glutamatergic presynaptic cell, incorporating NO.

4. Discuss the ways that each of the following could contribute to inhibition of a neuron:
   a. Change in threshold
   b. Change in resting membrane potential relative to threshold
   c. Increased chloride or potassium permeability: change in potential, change in conductance
   d. Presynaptic inhibition.

■ REFERENCES AND ADDITIONAL READINGS

Aidley DJ: *The physiology of excitable cells*, ed 4, Cambridge, 1998, Cambridge University Press.

Akabas MH, Kaufmann C, Archdeacon P, et al: Identification of acetylcholine receptor-channel-lining residues in the entire M2 segment of the α-subunit, *Neuron* 13:919-927, 1994.

Alberts B, Bray D, Lewis J, et al: *Molecular biology of the cell*, ed 4, New York, 2001, Garland Publishing.

Brown D: M-currents: an update, *Trends Neurosci* 11:294-299, 1988.

Brown DA, Adams PR: Muscarinic suppression of a novel voltage-sensitive K$^+$ current in a vertebrate neurone, *Nature* 283:673-676, 1980.

Choi DW: Calcium and exitotoxic neuronal injury, *Ann NY Acad Sci* 747:162-171, 1994.

Cooper JR, Bloom FE, Roth RH: *The biochemical basis of neuropharmacology*, ed 7, Oxford, 1996, Oxford University Press.

Cowan WM, Sudhof TC, Stevens CF: *Synapses,* Baltimore, 2000, Johns Hopkins University Press.

Gilman AG: Nobel lecture: G proteins and regulation of adenylyl cyclase, *Biosci Rep* 15:65-97, 1995.

Hamm HE: The many faces of G protein signaling, *J Biol Chem* 273:669-672, 1998.

Hebb DO: *The organization of behavior: a neuropsychological theory,* New York, 1949, John S. Wiley.

Hille B: Modulation of ion-channel function by G-protein-coupled receptors, *Trends Neurosci* 17:531-536, 1994.

Hollmann M, Heinemann S: Cloned glutamate receptors, *Annu Rev Neurosci* 17:31-108, 1994.

Huganir RL, Greengard P: Regulation of neurotransmitter receptor desensitization by protein phosphorylation, *Neuron* 5:555-567, 1990.

Jessell TM, Kandel ER: Synaptic transmission: a bi-directional and self-modifiable form of cell-cell communication, *Cell* 72(suppl):1-30, 1993.

Kandel ER, Schwartz JH, Jessell TM: *Principles of neural science*, ed 4, New York, 2000, McGraw-Hill.

Karlin A, Akabas MH: Toward a structural basis for the function of nicotinic acetylcholine receptors and their cousins, *Neuron* 15:1231-1244, 1995.

Kennedy MB: Second messengers and neuronal function. In Hall ZW (ed): *An introduction to molecular neurobiology*, Sunderland, Mass, 1992, Sinauer Associates, pp 207-246.

Kennedy MB: Signal processing machines at the postsynaptic density, *Science* 290:750–754, 2000.

Kuhse J, Betz H, Kirsch J: The inhibitory glycine receptor: architecture, synaptic localization, and molecular pathology of a postsynaptic ion channel complex, *Curr Opin Neurobiol* 5:318–323, 1995.

Levitan IB, Kaczmarek LK: *Neuromodulation: the biochemical control of neuronal excitability,* Oxford, 1987, Oxford University Press.

Logothetis DE, Kurachi Y, Galper J, et al: The βγ subunits of GTP-binding proteins activate the muscarinic K+ channel in heart, *Nature* 325:321–326, 1987.

Masu M, Tanabe Y, Tsuchida K, et al: Sequence and expression of a metabotropic glutamate receptor, *Nature* 349:760–765, 1991.

Moriyoshi K, Masu M, Ishii T, et al: Molecular cloning and characterization of the rat NMDA receptor, *Nature* 354: 31–37, 1991.

Nestler EJ, Hyman SE, Malenka RC: *Molecular neuropharmacology: a foundation for clinical neuroscience,* New York, 2001, McGraw-Hill.

Nicoll RA, Malenka RC, Kauer JA: Functional comparison of neurotransmitter receptor subtypes in mammalian central nervous system, *Physiol Rev* 70:513–565, 1990.

Niemann H, Blasi J, Jahn R: Clostridial neurotoxins: new toxins for dissecting exocytosis, *Trends Cell Biol* 4:179–185, 1994.

Noda M, Furutani Y, Takahashi H, et al: Cloning and sequence analysis of calf cDNA and human genomic DNA encoding α-subunit precursor of muscle acetylcholine receptor, *Nature* 305:818–823, 1983.

Noda M, Takahashi H, Tanabe T, et al: Structural homology of *Torpedo californica* acetylcholine receptor subunits, *Nature* 302:528–523, 1983.

Ross EM: G proteins and receptors in neuronal signaling. In Hall ZW (ed): *An introduction to molecular neurobiology,* Sunderland, Mass, 1992, Sinauer Associates, pp 181–206.

Siegelbaum SA, Tsien RW: Modulation of gated ion channels as a mode of neurotransmitter action, *Trends Neurosci* 6:307–313, 1983.

Smith GB, Olsen RW: Functional domains of GABA$_A$ receptors, *Trends Pharmacol Sci* 16:162–168, 1995.

Stahl SM: *Essential psychopharmacology,* ed 2, Cambridge, 2000, Cambridge University Press.

Strader CD, Fong TM, Tota MR, et al: Structure and function of G-protein-coupled receptors, *Annu Rev Biochem* 63: 101–132, 1994.

Unwin N: Neurotransmitter action: opening of ligand-gated ion channels, *Cell* 72(suppl):31–41, 1993.

Wickman KD, Clapham DE: G-protein regulation of ion channels, *Curr Opin Neurobiol* 5:278–285, 1995.

Wo ZG, Oswald RE: Unraveling the modular design of glutamate-gated ion channels, *Trends Neurosci* 18:161–168, 1995.

Zigmond MJ, Bloom FE, Roberts JL, et al (eds): *Fundamental neuroscience,* New York, 1999, Academic Press.

■ ANSWERS

Text Questions

1. An ionophore is the hydrophilic channel formed by a group of proteins that span the lipoidal membrane. It forms a pathway for ions to cross the membrane. The conformation of the proteins and the charge and intermolecular spacing of amino acid residues of the proteins determine the selectivity of the channel. Technically, the channels formed by the proteins of voltage-gated channels could also be called *ionophores,* but this term is used exclusively to refer to the channel formed by directly-gated ligand channels. Because any ion channel ultimately has the same task of differentiating among ions that can pass through it, it should not be too surprising that channels selective for a particular ion, such as K+, do share molecular similarities, regardless of their gating mechanism.

2. Five (2α, β, γ, and δ). The α subunits bind acetylcholine; each α subunit binds one molecule of ACh and each α subunit must be occupied for the channel to open. Thus two molecules of ACh are needed to open the channel. All five subunits contribute to forming the ionophore.

3. Reversal potential is a value of membrane potential at which an applied transmitter causes no change in potential but still causes an increase in conductance to ions. It represents the level of membrane potential at which there is no net movement of ions through a ligand-gated channel because the electrochemical gradients on all permeant ions for that channel are exactly balanced, equal, and opposite to one another.

4. $ACh_r = RT/F \ln \{(P_{Na}[Na^+]_o + P_K[K^+]_o) /$
$\quad\quad (P_{Na}[Na^+]_i + P_K[K^+]_i)\}$
$\quad = 61 \log_{10} \{(150 + 5) / (15 + 125)\}$
$\quad = 61 \log_{10} \{1.107\}$
$\quad = 61 \{0.044\}$
$\quad = + 2.7$ mV.

Depending on the preparation and the exact concentrations of Na^+ and K^+ ions, the value of ACh_r may vary a bit but is usually always in the range of –15 to + 15 mV. In the examples used in Figures 7-2 and 7-3, a value of –10 mV was used for Ach_r. The reason the value of ACh_r was different is that E_{Na} and E_K were different, and that is because the intracellular and extracellular concentrations of Na^+ and K^+ were slightly different in the two cases.

5. The NMDA receptor is unique because it is blocked at normal resting potentials by the presence of Mg^{++} ions in the mouth of the channel's extracellular surface. Cationic currents cannot move through the channel until the Mg^{++} ions are displaced from the channel opening. This is accomplished by membrane depolarization, which is induced by activation of nearby AMPA receptors.

6. At the resting potential, the outward concentration gradient on K^+ ions is slightly larger than the inward negative electrical gradient. If a transmitter opens K^+-selective channels, the net electrochemical gradient would allow K^+ ions to leave the cell. Outward movement of these positive charges would make the inside of the neuron more negative. Thus the membrane moves in the hyperpolarizing direction toward E_K and away from threshold when K^+ channels are opened.

7. Opening $GABA_A$ Cl^- channels in a membrane clamped at –40 mV would result in a large inward flow of Cl^- ions. Recall that the concentration gradient on these ions is directed inward (like it is for Na^+ ions). The inward movement of Cl^- ions down this gradient is prevented by the large negative internal resting potential. If we reduce this electrical gradient by depolarizing the neuron from rest to –40 mV, the electrical driving force repelling inward Cl^- movements is reduced. Thus there would be an influx of Cl^- ionic current. In a current-clamped neuron, this Cl^- influx would produce a large IPSP (see Figure 7-5, *B*).

8. Metabotropic receptors constitute a single large protein that has seven membrane spanning α-helices. (They are not multimeric nor do they form ion channels.) The binding site for small-molecule transmitters is buried among α-helical coils relatively deep within the outer leaflet of the membrane. Cytoplasmic loops, especially the one between helices 5 and 6, are required for binding to the α subunit of the G-protein. The carboxyl tail of the receptor is on the cytoplasmic side of the membrane and can be phosphorylated.

9. G-proteins are composed of three subunits: the α subunit, which is also the subunit with the guanosine binding site; and the $\beta\gamma$ subunits, which are tightly bound to one another and anchor the trimeric complex to the inner leaflet of the membrane. With activation of a receptor, the α subunit binds to the receptor and, with assistance from the $\beta\gamma$ dimer, exchanges GDP for GTP. This exchange then permits the α subunit to move laterally in the membrane and bind to a specific "primary effector protein," typically an enzyme that then initiates a cascade of biochemical reactions. The G-

protein complex thus serves to transduce information from a receptor to other reactants in a cell.

10. Adenylyl cyclase produces cAMP; phospholipase C produces IP_3 and DAG; phospholipase A_2 produces arachidonic acid.

11. cAMP initiates activity in phosphokinases A (PKA); IP_3 causes the release of Ca^{++} from intracellular stores; DAG activates phospholipase C (PKC); arachidonic acid is broken down to generate numerous metabolites; Ca^{++} ions can interact with calmodulin to induce CaM-kinase

12. Ca^{++} ions are required for transmitter release, and they can directly influence the activity of some channel proteins. For example, they can turn on voltage-gated K^+ channels (so-called Ca^{++}-dependent K^+ channels). They can also enter the cell through voltage-gated Ca^{++} channels as part of the action potential current in some neurons and muscle cells. Ca^{++} ions are also required for muscle contraction and can regulate inactivation properties of some voltage-gated Ca^{++} channels. They also play a direct role in stabilizing the membrane potential by adding to the ionic strength of the extracellular fluid: too few divalent ions and the membrane becomes destabilized, threshold is lowered, and cells become too excitable; too many divalent ions and the opposite happens. Ca^{++} is extraordinarily important to the well being and homeostasis of excitable cells.

13. The slow EPSP seen in the postganglionic neuron would disappear because atropine blocked the mAChR causing this potential change. Only the fast EPSPs would remain.

14. The transmembrane ionic current carried through ligand-gated channels is led away from the site of transmitter action, spreading along the RC circuitry of the membrane. For example, the influx of Na^+ ions at the site of an opened cationic channel represents a brief pulse of positivity into the cell that will repel nearby K^+ ions that will move away through r_i and up to the membrane r_m-c_m network (see Chapter 3). Taking all those r_m's together, we can imagine that they might represent the overall resistance of the total membrane at rest. The total membrane resistance can be thought of as the "input resistance" of the neuron, R_i. The current produced by the transmitter, I_t, passes through R_i and creates a voltage change, V_t, the synaptic potential (by Ohm's law). If we lowered R_i by opening other channels (conductance increase), then I_t will produce a smaller V_t. The current spreading away from the site of I_t initiation can pass through the membrane via low-resistance open channels instead of going through r_m–c_m. Conversely, if typically open channels were closed, this could lead to an increase in R_i, and PSPs generated by the same I_t would be larger.

15. Reducing the resting potassium conductance will allow the membrane potential to move a little closer to E_{Na}. It is that simple if you remember the "golden rule": the membrane potential moves toward the equilibrium potential of the ion to which it is more permeable.

16. A presynaptic neuron makes a conventional synaptic connection with a postsynaptic neuron and produces an EPSP in the postsynaptic cell. A different neuron (the "modulator") sends an axon to end on the presynaptic ending of the first axon,

forming an axo-axonic synapse. The modulatory axon ending releases a transmitter onto the presynaptic terminal that induces some change in that terminal so that less transmitter is released. This reduction in transmitter release by the presynaptic axon will cause the EPSP in the postsynaptic cell to be smaller. The postsynaptic neuron has experienced a form of inhibition in the sense that it received less excitatory input than it otherwise would. Inhibition of this kind, that is, reduction in postsynaptic excitation produced by alterations in the presynaptic axon induced by a third cell, is called *presynaptic inhibition* (the postsynaptic cell is inhibited by some change in the presynaptic neuron).

■ POST-TEST

1. GABA released by the presynaptic axon will cause inhibition in the postsynaptic cell because there are GABA receptors in the postsynaptic neuron. If they were $GABA_A$ receptors, the GABA would drive the postsynaptic membrane potential toward E_{Cl}. The GABAergic terminal membrane has $GABA_B$ receptors in it. Some of these autoreceptors will be activated by the GABA released from this same terminal. The $GABA_B$ receptors, working through a G_i-protein, can have one or more of the following effects on the terminal: decrease g_{Ca}; inhibit adenylyl cyclase, thus reducing cAMP levels; or increase g_K. Each of these effects could cause a reduction in release of the GABA transmitter from the terminal. If less GABA is released, then the postsynaptic IPSP will be smaller and the postsynaptic cell will be less inhibited. This is a type of homosynaptic facilitation—obviously the cell is more excited than it was when the IPSPs were larger. A decrease in g_{Ca}

obviously means that less Ca^{++} would enter the presynaptic terminal through voltage-gated Ca^{++} channels when the action potential occurred. A reduction in $[Ca^{++}]_i$ will have a significant impact on vesicle release (remember synaptotagmin). Because cAMP plays a role in the biochemical events involved in release (CaM-K, as well as PKA, regulate synapsin binding to neurofilaments, for example), reducing cAMP will interfere with that process. Lowering $[Ca^{++}]_i$ would also reduce the amount of available CaM-K. An increase in g_K could speed the repolarization of the action potential, reducing the overall duration of the spike. Because the terminal is depolarized for a shorter period, fewer voltage-gated calcium channels will be opened, or the ones that are opened will close sooner. Thus less Ca^{++} will enter the terminal, so less transmitter will be released.

2. Blocking voltage-gated K^+ currents (reducing g_K) would slow action potential repolarization. The action potential duration would be increased: more Ca^{++} ions enter the terminal and more transmitter is released.

3. Glutamate released from the presynaptic terminal first activates ionotropic AMPA receptors, producing fast EPSPs. These EPSPs summate and depolarize the postsynaptic neuron adequately to remove the Mg^{++} block of NMDA receptors. This opening now lets Ca^{++} ions in through the cationic ionophore. The Ca^{++} binds calmodulin, and the Ca-calmodulin complex activates NOS, which now produces NO. The NO diffuses out of the postsynaptic cell, across the synaptic cleft, and into the presynaptic terminal where it stimulates the enzyme guanylyl cyclase. The guanylyl

cyclase catalyzes the production of cGMP, which then facilitates release of glutamate from the presynaptic terminal. Greater release of glutamate would only reinforce this cycle.

4. a. Inhibition, in general, means a decrease in the probability that a cell will fire an action potential or that there is a decrease in the excitability of the cell. Inhibition is most commonly discussed in terms of the typical way it occurs in nerve cells, by the production of IPSPs. However, there are numerous ways a cell may be inhibited. IPSPs have complex mechanisms of action, and cells can be effectively inhibited by removing or reducing excitatory inputs (presynaptic inhibition). Anything that increases threshold will inhibit a cell. Earlier it was mentioned that divalent ion concentrations can influence threshold by their stabilizing effects on the membrane field potential. Raising divalent ion concentrations can indeed make cells less excitable or raise their threshold, but such changes in divalent ion concentration do not occur under physiological conditions. Most natural events in the brain do not directly affect threshold, but numerous "artificial" factors do. For example, cooling raises threshold directly, as do local anesthetics, nerve compression, and some toxins (like tetrodotoxin). Strictly speaking, anything that reduces excitability increases threshold, because the two are inversely related. Thus the factors discussed below, which do depress excitability, can be thought of as raising threshold.

   b. If the cell's membrane potential is moved in the depolarizing direction, the cell is more excitable because it is approaching the level of membrane potential designated as threshold—the potential at which voltage-gated sodium channels initiate the action potential. Anytime the membrane potential is moved in the hyperpolarizing direction, more negative than the resting potential, the cell is inhibited, if for no other reason, simply because the potential now "has farther to go" before it reaches threshold. Thus anything that drives the membrane potential in the negative direction will inhibit the cell. An applied negative internal current (cathode) or external anode (positive) will hyperpolarize the cell. Any transmitter or drug that increases the conductance of the membrane to an ion that has an equilibrium potential more negative than the resting potential will hyperpolarize and inhibit the cell.

   c. Because E_K and E_{Cl} are normally more negative than the resting potential, increasing the permeability of the membrane to either of these ions will inhibit the cell. Even if E_{Cl} is less negative than the resting potential, increasing the permeability of the membrane to Cl^- will move the membrane potential to E_{Cl} but not beyond or any closer to threshold. Even if the resting potential, E_K and E_{Cl} were all the same value, increasing g_K or g_{Cl} would still inhibit the cell: not because the membrane moves more negative, but because conductance has been increased (lowered membrane resistance). A reduction in membrane resistance will tend to decrease the amplitude of EPSPs because their currents will be shunted through the lowered membrane resistance.

d. Presynaptic inhibition is another means of inhibiting cells, whereby modulatory inputs to presynaptic terminals that are excitatory to a postsynaptic cell can induce changes in the presynaptic terminal that cause a reduction in the amount of excitatory transmitter released. This will reduce the amplitude of the EPSP, making the postsynaptic cell less excited than it would otherwise have been.

Index

Page references in *italic* indicate figures, and page numbers followed by t indicate tables.